KU-277-141

Royal Liverpool University Hospital – Staff Library (Education Centre)

Please return or renew, on or before the last date below. A fine is payable on late returned items. Books may be recalled after one week for the use of another reader. Books may be renewed by telephone : 0151-706-2248

A Colour Atlas of **Foot** and **Ankle** Disorders

For Audrey and Stephen Edmonds, Julien and William Foster, Antonia Wray, and Andrew and Hilary Reid, with love and thanks.

For Elsevier:

Commissioning Editor: Robert Edwards
Development Editor: Rebecca Gleave
Project Manager: Jess Thompson
Designer: Stewart Larking

A COLOUR ATLAS OF
Foot and Ankle Disorders

By
Alethea V. M. Foster
BA(Hons) PGCE DPodM MChS SRCh
Formerly Lead Clinical Specialist Podiatrist,
King's College Hospital NHS Trust,
London, UK.

and
Michael E. Edmonds
MD FRCP
Consultant Physician, Diabetic Foot Clinic,
King's College Hospital NHS Trust,
London, UK.

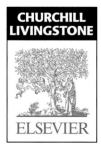

Edinburgh London New York Oxford Philadelphia St Louis Sydney Toronto 2007

CHURCHILL
LIVINGSTONE

© 2007, Elsevier Limited. All rights reserved.

No part of this publication may be reproduced, stored in a retrieval system, or transmitted in any form or by any means, electronic, mechanical, photocopying, recording or otherwise, without the prior permission of the Publishers. Permissions may be sought directly from Elsevier's Health Sciences Rights Department, 1600 John F. Kennedy Boulevard, Suite 1800, Philadelphia, PA 19103-2899, USA: phone: (+1) 215 239 3804; fax: (+1) 215 239 3805; or, e-mail: *healthpermissions@elsevier.com*. You may also complete your request on-line via the Elsevier homepage (http://www.elsevier.com), by selecting 'Support and contact' and then 'Copyright and Permission'.

First published 2007

ISBN 978 0443 102073
British Library Cataloguing in Publication Data
A catalogue record for this book is available from the British Library

Library of Congress Cataloging in Publication Data
A catalog record for this book is available from the Library of Congress

Knowledge and best practice in this field are constantly changing. As new research and experience broaden our knowledge, changes in practice, treatment and drug therapy may become necessary or appropriate. Readers are advised to check the most current information provided (i) on procedures featured or (ii) by the manufacturer of each product to be administered, to verify the recommended dose or formula, the method and duration of administration, and contraindications. It is the responsibility of the practitioner, relying on their own experience and knowledge of the patient, to make diagnoses, to determine dosages and the best treatment for each individual patient, and to take all appropriate safety precautions.
To the fullest extent of the law, neither the publisher nor the editors assumes any liability for any injury and/or damage.

The ***Publisher***

Printed in China

ELSEVIER your source for books, journals and multimedia in the health sciences
www.elsevierhealth.com

Working together to grow
libraries in developing countries

www.elsevier.com | www.bookaid.org | www.sabre.org

ELSEVIER   BOOK AID International   Sabre Foundation

The publisher's policy is to use **paper manufactured from sustainable forests**

Contents

All the images in this colour atlas are of patients from the Foot Clinic at King's College Hospital NHS Trust. Our busy, multidisciplinary foot team is made up of physicians, podiatrists, nurses, surgeons and orthotists. The clinic is open for 5 full days a week, offering assessment and care-planning appointments for local and tertiary referrals, and routine follow-up appointments for people in need of continuing care.

The King's catchment area has interesting contrasts: it includes the local "Millionaires' Row" in Dulwich Village, and also areas of some of the greatest inner-city social deprivation in the United Kingdom, as seen in Camberwell and Peckham. Affluence, poverty and ignorance side by side, within a few hundred yards of each other; Caucasians, Afro-Caribbeans and Asians, make for an interesting mix of foot problems.

Referral to the Foot Clinic comes from general practitioners, other community health-care professionals (including practice nurses, district nurses and podiatrists), departments within King's such as Accident and Emergency, and hospitals throughout the United Kingdom. The King's Foot Clinic also acts as an Accident and Emergency department to our own foot patients and the local population, as well as being a centre for teaching, research and clinical trials.

Throughout our writing, we have only ever described medical conditions of which we have first-hand experience, having seen, treated and followed them in our own Foot Clinic. For this reason, readers should be warned that in this book there may be some gaps or omissions of interesting and relevant foot conditions, which are excluded solely because they have never presented to us. We considered borrowing pictures from colleagues and our publisher to fill these gaps, but felt that inclusion of conditions where there is lack of first-hand practical experience will always result in a less useful, less practical, and far less authoritative text. Our aim has always been to speak and teach with the conviction that can only be based on long-term and immediate clinical experience.

However, we hope that the reader will find compensations for any gaps within these pages, for we include some very rare conditions, including a case of human plectophomella chromomycosis, and exotic gems such as mycosis fungoides, pasteurella multocida and vibrio vulnificus, along with more common conditions. We have also included a few pictures of hands, legs and faces in addition to feet and ankles in order to illustrate important features of systemic diseases.

We hope, overall, that this book will be a useful guide to the diagnosis and management of both common and rare conditions. For this is, above all, a colour atlas with a very *practical focus* and intent. We want to get across to our readers the flavour of working in a pioneering establishment, and the excitement of encountering patients in the real world, where things happen unexpectedly, diagnosis and treatment are sometimes very challenging, clinics are crowded, and clinicians are overstretched. The pictures in this book of feet are not staid or routine: these are the patients who were seen amid the hustle and bustle, and hurly burly of daily clinical life. Up to 50 patients can pass through the King's Foot Clinic in a single morning, nearly all of whom fall into the high-risk category and many of whom present as extremely challenging emergencies.

We organize and run a Foot Clinic because the foot is so important. The foot can be a shining light in the darkness, a beacon which is an important illuminator or indicator of multi-system disease. The foot can direct the careful observer towards the specific body systems affected by diseases that may not previously have been diagnosed. The pictures in this book represent a selection of interesting cases that we have seen. They represent the spectrum of presentations that the practitioner might reasonably expect to meet and manage. Our previous publications have been solely about the problems of the diabetic foot. However, over the past 25 years we have also obtained experience of numerous foot problems that are not related to diabetes or arise in non-diabetic patients, and these are the patients covered in this book.

The approach in this book is very practical. We describe, using pictures, the appearance of the patient at presentation adding small details about the patient that will, we hope, bring the picture to life, illuminating a real person with a real foot problem and the things that need to be done to help that patient. Notes are minimal but some highlighted points will include such areas as: problems of differential diagnosis, how the foot was examined, what investigations were performed to clarify the situation and useful tips as to management (how to tell if treatment is succeeding and the outcomes to be expected).

Where the treatments offered fall into our area of expertise and are unusual or non-routine, then we will sometimes comment briefly upon them; however, we do not discuss treatments or conditions that fall into the realms of other specialities, apart from mentioning the need for referral onwards. Any Foot Clinic will always need to develop close links with other departments to ensure rapid and appropriate treatment of all patients. Overall, outcomes can often be very good, as shown in Figures 1A and B.

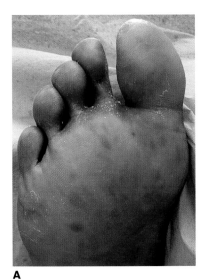 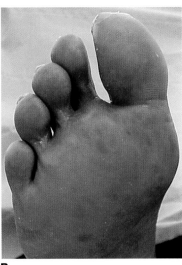

A **B**

1A Good outcomes with regular care from a multidisciplinary Foot Clinic. Outcomes can be very good with regular foot care. This diabetic patient presented aged 22 years with indolent neuropathic ulceration. This healed after a 5-week hospital admission for bed rest and antibiotics. **A** was taken 10 years later. The foot was still intact, and the patient was married and leading an active life. **1B** The same patient 20 years after he was first seen in the Foot Clinic, and the foot is still intact. The patient has attended the clinic at monthly intervals for removal of callus over the site of previous ulceration. He wears bespoke shoes with cradled insoles and checks his feet every day.

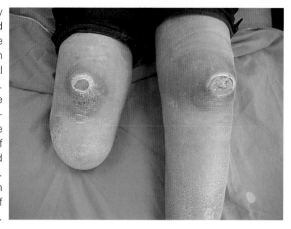

2 Acquired immune deficiency syndrome (AIDS) and neuropathic ulceration of the knees. This young man with AIDS developed peripheral neuropathy and foot ulceration. After an episode of severe sepsis, he underwent a below-knee amputation. He was unable to wear a prosthesis because of fluctuant swelling, and crawled around the house on his knees. He presented 3 weeks later with infected neuropathic ulceration of the knees.

This book is designed to be of use to all healthcare professionals encountering patients with foot problems, be they in the hospital or community setting. It is a book about real patients in real situations, as indicated in Figure 2.

Further reading

Readers with a particular interest in diabetes are referred to our previous publications:

Foster AVM. The Podiatric Assessment and Management of the Diabetic Foot. Churchill Livingstone, 2006.

Edmonds M, Foster A. Managing the Diabetic Foot, 2nd edn. Blackwell Science, 2005.

Edmonds M, Foster A, Sanders L. A Practical Manual of Diabetic Foot Care, Blackwell Science, 2004.

We are grateful to colleagues past and present, who include: Simon Fraser, Huw Walters, Mary Blundell, Cathy Eaton, Mark Greenhill, Susie Spencer, Maureen McColgan-Bates, Mel Doxford, Sally Wilson, Adora Hatrapal, E Maelor Thomas, Mick Morris, John Philpott-Howard, Jim Wade, Andrew Hay, Robert Lewis, Anne-Marie Ryan, Irina Mantey, Robert Hills, Rachel Ben-Salem, Muriel Buxton-Thomas, Mazin Al-Janabi, Dawn Hurley, Stephanie Amiel, Stephen Thomas, Daniela Pitei, Paul Baskerville, Anthony Giddings, Irving Benjamin, Mark Myerson, Paul Sidhu, Joydeep Sinha, Patricia Wallace, Gillian Cavell, Lesley Boys, Magdi Hanna, Sue Peat, Colin Roberts, David Goss, Colin Deane, Sue Snowdon, Ana Grenfell, Tim Cundy, Pat Ascott, Lindis Richards, Kate Spicer, Debbie Broome, Liz Hampton, Timothy Jemmott, Michelle Buckley, Rosalind Phelan, Maggie Boase, Maria Back, Avril Witherington, Daniel Rajan, Hisham Rashid, Ghulam Mufti, Karen Fairbairn, Ian Eltringham, Nina Petrova, Lindy Begg, Barbara Wall, Mark O'Brien, Sacha Andrews, Barry Pike, Jane Preece, Briony Sloper, Christian Pankhurst, Jim Beaumont, Matthew McShane, Cheryl Clark, Marcello Perez, Nicholas Cooley, Paul Bains, Patricia Yerbury, Charlotte Biggs, Anna Korzon Burakowska, David Ross, Jason Wilkins, David Evans, Carol Gayle, David Hopkins, Keith Jones, Bob Edmondson, Enid Joseph, Karen Reid, David Williams, Doris Agyemang-Duah, Jennifer Tremlett, Venu Kavarthapu, Om Lahori and Mark Phillips and two great stalwarts of the Foot Clinic, Peter Watkins and the late David Pyke. The Podiatry Managers and Community Podiatrists from Lambeth, Southwark and Lewisham have also contributed greatly to the work of the Foot Clinic at King's over many years.

We are particularly grateful for the advice of the members of the Dermatology Department, Anthony du Vivier, Daniel Creamer, Claire Fuller, Elisabeth Higgins and Sarah MacFarlane.

We also are also thankful to Audrey and Stephen Edmonds, and Nina Petrova for technical help with the production of the manuscript.

We give special thanks to Yvonne Bartlett, Alex Dionysiou, David Langdon, Lucy Wallace and Moira Lovell from the Department of Medical Photography at King's.

We are also grateful to Rebecca Gleave our Development Editor and Robert Edwards, our Commissioning Editor for their patience and encouragement.

Acknowledgements

Inspection

Inspection begins when the patient enters the Foot Clinic. It is important for the clinician to observe the gait when the patient is walking in, and to note the presence of any walking aids or a wheelchair. The shoes and hose should be removed and examined before the feet are inspected: valuable clues may be revealed by wear marks and state of repair of shoes and socks. It is also important to remove anything that is preventing full inspection of the feet and legs, including dressings, topical substances such as talcum powder, and dirt. Traditional folk remedies, such as henna, may have been applied topically to wounds, which can often render diagnosis more difficult because the wound is masked or the surface is stained.

An important aspect of the foot inspection for the clinician is to consider the way the patient presented, which may reveal valuable information about the relevant background, including social, economic and psychological problems. The photographs of patients shown below illustrate this.

A common problem of differential diagnosis is shown in Figure 3. This diabetic patient presented with a red, hot, swollen foot. Is this cellulitis, Charcot's osteoarthropathy or gout? What investigations were performed to clarify the situation and come to the correct diagnosis?

It is essential to catch problems early. Figure 4 shows a patient with an infected breakdown on the distal part of a previously fully-healed skin graft. The clinician needs to explore the cause of the breakdown, and to consider aspects of preventing further problems as well as commencing rapid and effective treatment of the existing problem.

The clinician needs to be aware that a careful search for subtle early warning signs that all is not well is essential if he wishes to "nip" the pathological process "in the bud". It is only by detecting signs that things are going wrong that the clinician will be able to keep control of the situation, and prevent avoidable problems from getting out of hand (see Fig. 5A, where the 4th toe is swollen and Fig. 5B, where the 4th toe is deteriorating rapidly when no action is taken).

It is also essential that clinicians never underestimate the importance of recording each day's findings carefully, as they can be used as a baseline against which future changes can be measured, as shown in Figures 6A, B and C, which show a patient's foot deteriorating when he fails to follow advice and then improving after he agrees to follow advice and rest the foot.

When a patient first presents at the Foot Clinic, both feet are inspected and compared, as in Figure 7. This comparison of the feet and lower limbs is essential; without it, significant pathology may be missed. The colour of the foot, the wound bed and surrounding tissue is a valuable aid to diagnosis. Colour change may be intrinsic, as in the redness of cellulitis, or extrinsic, as shown in Figures 8, 9 and 10, where staining is due to henna, potassium permanganate and Pseudomonas aeruginosa infection, respectively.

Infection may lead to changes in the colour of the wound bed, as shown in Figure 11, where the toe is infected and the nail bed is grey. When tissue is discoloured and opaque it may need to be removed, as shown in Figures 12A and B, which show a heel pressure ulcer pre and post debridement. Figure 12C shows an orthosis to prevent heel ulceration. The presence of pain is important and Figure 13 shows a painful, discoloured ischaemic heel.

Changes in the shape of a foot or part of a foot are usually significant. In Figure 14, the patient has developed a bursa over his hallux valgus, while in Figure 15, the "sausage-like" appearance of this toe, with redness and fusiform swelling, is due to osteomyelitis.

The presence of oedema or wrinkles, other skin abnormalities (including dry skin, atrophy, thickening of nails or skin, callus, cracking), or specific lesions such as blisters and ulcers should be noted, and any factors that may mask the problem should be taken into account; appearances may often be deceptive, as in Figure 16, where the foot is masked with talcum powder. A careful examination will include sites between the toes; Figure 17 shows tinea pedis and Figure 18 an infected interdigital ulcer as examples of lesions that will be missed if the area between the toes is overlooked.

The clinician should enquire about concurrent health problems, which may render a certain diagnosis more likely, and always look for factors that will give away other problems. Figure 19 is the foot of a patient in end-stage renal failure; other examples are of people with social problems, neglected feet, feet in old age, and feet of people with psychological problems (Fig. 20).

Palpation

It is essential to assess the patient for the presence of peripheral vascular disease. The pedal pulses should be palpated, and if they are weak or absent then a small hand-held Doppler can be used to measure the ankle brachial pressure index. If the feet are particularly cold or warm then this should be noted: Figure 21A shows a foot that was cold because of acute ischaemia and Figure 21B shows marks left after removal of an overly tight sock from an ischaemic leg. If one foot is more than 2°C hotter than the other foot and the patient has peripheral neuropathy, then the problem may be acute Charcot's osteoarthropathy. Figure 22 shows the hot swollen foot with the dilated veins characteristic of a Charcot foot. The presence of pitting oedema, and the texture and consistency of tissues, should be palpated and noted. Joint mobility and range of movement (both active and passive) at particular joints should be assessed. Limitation of movement can lead to foot problems, as shown in Figures 23A and B, where the patient has hallux rigidus and has developed callus, shown pre and post debridement.

As in the visual inspection, comparison of the foot and leg with the contralateral foot and leg is always important when palpating the foot. It is essential to compare both feet and legs. If a skin thermometer is not available then the back of the hand is sufficiently sensitive to detect significant temperature disparities between the limbs.

Debridement

Surface appearances may be deceptive, and debridement can reveal the state of affairs. Before commencing debridement, it is essential to ascertain whether the foot is ischaemic. Figures 24A–E demonstrate the debridement of a healed ischaemic ulcer. Sometimes callus is amalgamated with toenail but should be removed carefully (Fig. 25). The depth of an ulcer can be revealed by probing (Fig. 26). Debridement reveals any undermining, and should lay open the wound, reveal the depth and remove surface necrosis (Figs 27A and B). The debridement of a neuropathic ulcer is shown in Figures 28A–E (see Chapter 4 on inspecting nails and examples of cutting back the nail to reveal the nail bed for inspection).

In addition to visual inspection and palpation, the clinician may rely on the other senses; she may smell odour in infection or neglected feet, her eyes may be stinging from ammonia present in wound miasma, and she may hear the crepitus of gas in severely infected tissues.

It is important to question the patient and the family when seeking the cause of an unusual problem. Figures 29A and B show a case of allergy to a Christmas tree. Family members can be encouraged to accompany the patient to the Foot Clinic. A careful eye should be kept out for social problems leading to foot trouble. Figure 30 is a case of rat bite and Figure 31 shows flesh fly maggots in a neglected foot. A friendly relaxed atmosphere is important, as those attending the clinic may be extremely anxious, as were the parents of the newborn baby with eczema shown in Figure 32.

The duration of any lesion, cause of the lesion and previous treatment of the lesion should always be ascertained. Figures 33A and B show early burns and late presenting burns.

Investigations

The Foot Clinic often needs to organise and perform investigations. X-rays may reveal a foreign body, as shown in Figure 34. The importance of correct views and timing for X-rays should not be underestimated and it is helpful to keep X-rays as a baseline against which future changes can be assessed. CT scans, MRI scans, microbiology specimens, Doppler examinations and blood tests etc. all have an important place in the armamentarium of the Foot Clinic.

Problems of differential diagnosis

Diagnosis of foot problems may not be easy. The differential diagnosis of a red foot, as shown in Figure 35, may include dermatitis or cellulitis or Charcot's osteoarthropathy (diagnosis was allergic contact dermatitis). The diagnosis of vasculitis (as seen in Fig. 36) can cause difficulties. Is Figure 37 showing malignancy or haemorrhage within an indolent pressure ulcer? Figure 38 shows pruritic and flaking skin; is the problem a fungal infection or dermatitis? Are the small non-blanching lesions shown in Figure 39 micro-emboli or vasculitis?

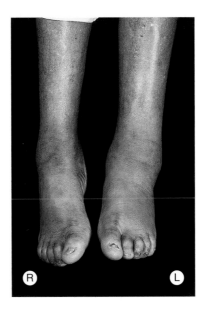

3 Red, hot, swollen foot. This is a problem of differential diagnosis. The patient had diabetes and peripheral neuropathy and presented with a red, hot, swollen left foot. The differential diagnosis included cellulitis, Charcot's osteoarthropathy and gout. Serum urate was normal, thus making gout unlikely. There was no obvious portal of entry or break in the skin, so infection was unlikely. An X-ray was normal but the diphosphonate bone scan showed increased uptake, confirming the diagnosis of Charcot's osteoarthropathy. He was treated in a total contact cast.

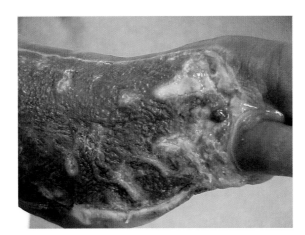

4 Infected skin graft. This patient underwent extensive debridement of an infected foot. When the wound had a good granulating bed it was grafted; the donor site was on the patient's thigh. Unfortunately the graft was not followed up regularly in a Foot Clinic. Callus was allowed to become so thick that parts of the graft broke down and became infected. All skin grafts on the foot should be checked regularly and any callus that develops should be sharp debrided by a podiatrist.

5A The 4th toe is pink and swollen and shows signs of infection. A collection of pus under the 4th metatarsal head had been previously drained.
5B The 4th toe is now dusky, indicating a relative oxygen deficit to the skin because of a septic arteritis reducing digital artery blood flow to the toe.

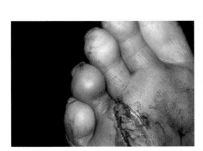

A

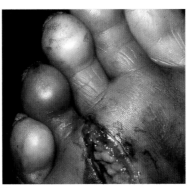

B

6A Friction burns leading to neuropathic ulceration. This is the foot of a young patient with diabetic neuropathy. He lay in the bath for 30 minutes, and then heard the telephone ringing, got out of the bath and ran to answer it. He felt that his foot problem was due to friction from his nylon carpet when he ran, with bare feet. The skin was macerated from soaking in the bath. The rough carpet abraded the delicate, macerated skin of his foot leading to friction burns and extensive desquamation and ulceration. Only one foot was affected and no other areas of his body were burnt. He denied resting the foot on the hot tap or hot water pipes. The foot was debrided and dressed and he was advised to rest it.

6B The same foot 11 days later. The patient felt, despite our advice, that resting the foot was not necessary and on return to the Foot Clinic the ulceration was far more extensive. He then agreed to take time off work. Antibiotics were prescribed.

6C The same foot after 16 more days have elapsed. He had been trying to rest and the toes and the forefoot ulcer have improved.

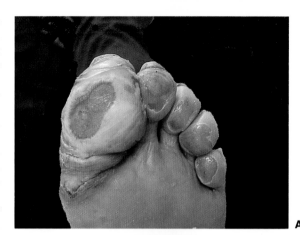

A

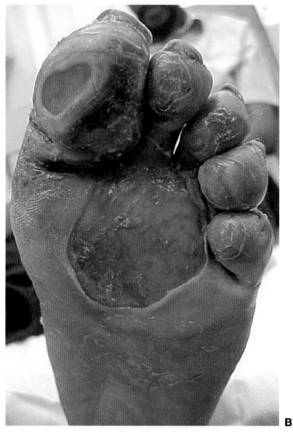

B

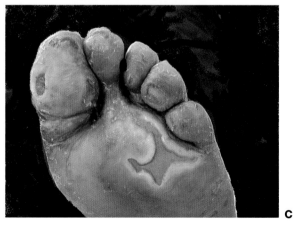

C

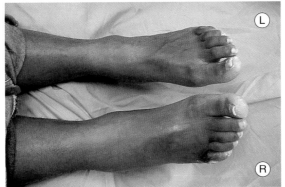
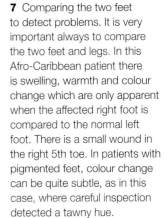

7 Comparing the two feet to detect problems. It is very important always to compare the two feet and legs. In this Afro-Caribbean patient there is swelling, warmth and colour change which are only apparent when the affected right foot is compared to the normal left foot. There is a small wound in the right 5th toe. In patients with pigmented feet, colour change can be quite subtle, as in this case, where careful inspection detected a tawny hue.

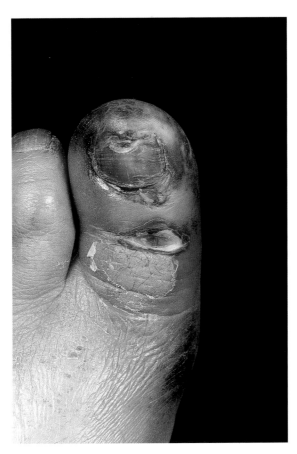

8 Henna staining masquerading as gangrene. A diabetic patient from North Africa was reported to have developed "gangrene". In fact, the black patches were caused by her having painted the foot with henna, which is a traditional folk remedy for wounds. Any topical application that stains the foot in this way can make it difficult to assess the foot.

9 Staining from potassium permanganate. This patient was prescribed potassium permanganate footbaths to treat a fungal infection. The strong solution of potassium permanganate had discoloured the skin and nails.

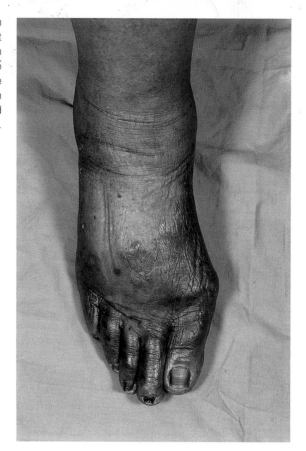

10 Pseudomonas aeruginosa infection. The discharge from this patient's ulcer had greenish discolouration and a fusty, musty odour reminiscent of mouse urine and suggestive of Pseudomonas aeruginosa infection. The dressing was heavily stained; the presence of Pseudomonas was confirmed on culture.

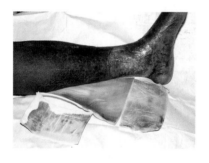

11 Infected nail bed. This patient presented with a cellulitic toe following a traumatic avulsion of the nail. Note the greyish discolouration of the nail bed, which is an early marker of severe infection. However, a recent application of liquid phenol to ablate the nail bed will also lead to grey discolouration.

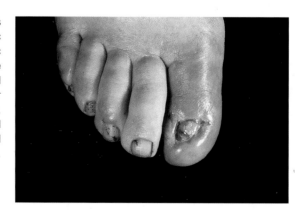

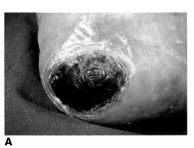

A

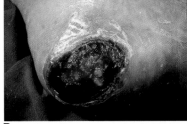

B

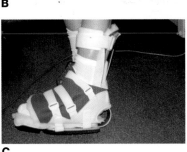

C

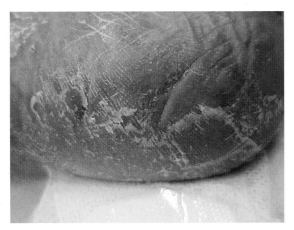

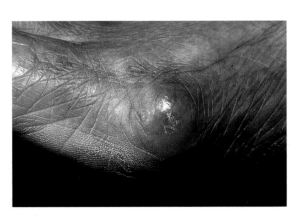

12A Heel necrosis. This patient presented with a patch of dry necrosis on the heel following a period of immobilization in bed. The pedal pulses were palpable. It can be difficult to ascertain the extent of the problem and the depth of the necrosis.

12B In this case, the foot was gently debrided, revealing a normal fat pad beneath the necrosis. The foot healed in a total contact cast.

12C Prevention is easier than cure; it should be mandatory for immobile, bed-bound patients to be given heel protection. A useful technique to relieve heel pressure is the Pressure Relieving Ankle Foot Orthosis (PRAFO).

13 Pain and discolouration in an ischaemic heel. This elderly patient complained of pain in the heel of 3 days' duration and was referred to the Foot Clinic as an emergency by his general practitioner. The ankle/brachial pressure index was 0.34. There was a small fissure on the heel associated with bluish discolouration. He underwent angioplasty and the foot improved.

14 Bursitis caused by an unsuitable shoe. This is bursitis associated with chronic pressure from a "pointy-toed" shoe, which led to inflammation and formation of an adventitious bursa over the 1st metatarsophalangeal joint. The problem resolved with a change to wider fitting shoes.

15 "Sausage toe" in osteomyelitis. This patient presented with redness and fusiform swelling of the toe of 2 months' duration. He complained of throbbing pain and there was a small discharging ulcer on the dorsum of the toe which probed to bone.

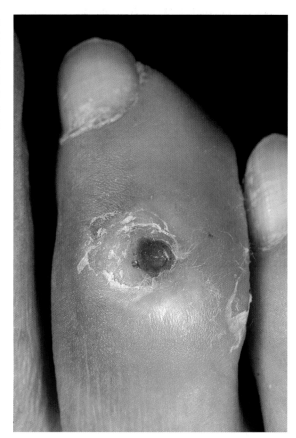

16 Overdose of talcum powder. This patient had to be advised to stop applying copious amounts of talcum powder to his feet. Excessive amounts of powder can cake between the toes causing soreness and can also mask signs such as discolouration or small breaks in the skin.

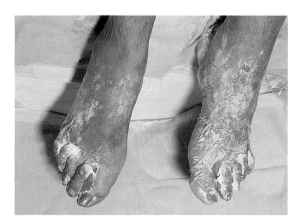

17 Inspecting for problems between the toes – tinea pedis. When examining the feet the interdigital areas should never be overlooked. Fungal infections are common, associated with rubbery white skin, furrowing and fissuring, and unpleasant odour.

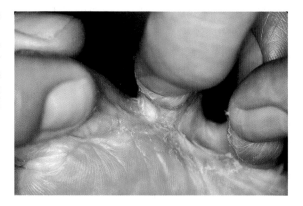

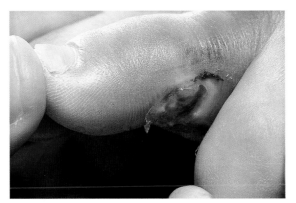

18 Infected interdigital ulcer. There is cellulitis of the toe and blue discolouration adjacent to the ulcer, indicating a lack of oxygen to the skin because of sepsis.

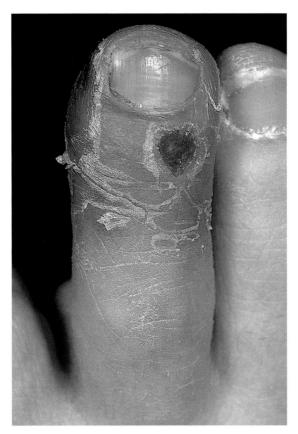

19 Early necrosis in the renal foot. This lesion appears to be small and trivial but is, in fact, an early presentation of necrosis in a patient in end-stage renal failure treated by renal transplantation. Renal patients have a great predisposition to develop necrosis (see Chapter 6 on metabolic disorders affecting the foot).

20 Dermatitis artefacta. This patient scratched the skin off her foot. She had a peripheral neuropathy.

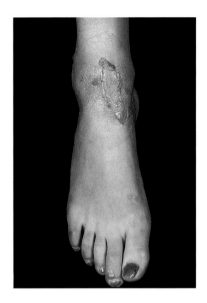

21A Acute ischaemia. This patient complained of severe pain and paraesthesiae. The foot was cold and blue. The patient was a heavy smoker.

21B The patient's socks were tight and had left marks on his leg. The pressure index was 0.21. This is a clinical emergency as without rapid vascular intervention the life and limb of the patient may be lost (see Chapter 3 for more ischaemic feet).

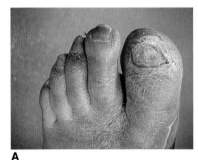

A

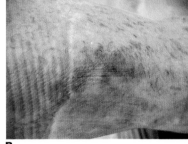

B

22 Early case of Charcot's osteoarthropathy. This condition can develop very rapidly. The patient presented with a hot, swollen foot 2 days after he came out of a plaster cast which was used to heal a neuropathic ulcer.

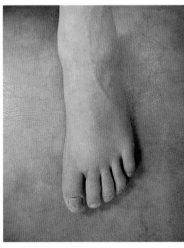
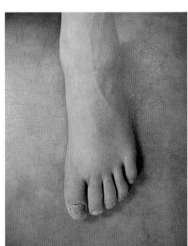

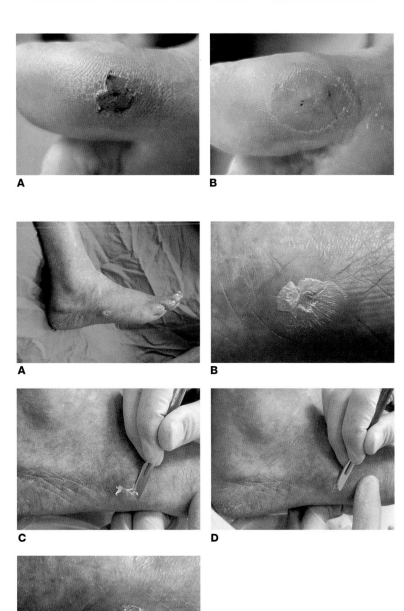

23A Hallux rigidus. This results from degenerative joint disease of the 1st metatarsophalangeal joint. Callus has developed on the medial plantar aspect of the interphalangeal joint and bleeding within the callus indicates that the patient is at risk of skin breakdown. **23B** This shows the same foot after debridement.

24A Healed ischaemic ulcer. There is a healed ischaemic ulcer overlaid by glassy callus on the lateral border of the foot. Ischaemic ulcers are commonly found on the vulnerable margins of the foot. **24B** Close-up view of the lesion. **24C** The podiatrist is gently removing overlying, glassy callus, with scalpel and forceps. **24D** Debriding debris and callus. **24E** The fully debrided healed ulcer.

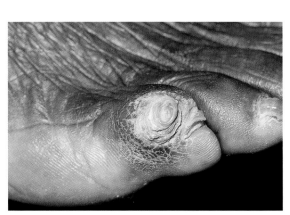

25 Callus amalgamated with nail. It can sometimes be difficult to tell where a callus ends and a nail begins. Nails that are associated with abnormal mechanical forces will thicken in the same way that skin develops excess keratin and thickens when subjected to pressure, shear or friction.

26 Probing ulcer with forceps. This method assesses undermining (where the wound "burrows" under apparently normal surrounding skin). The true dimensions of ulcers can be very deceptive and probing is a very useful technique for revealing the true extent of the problem. Medieval physicians would use a parsley stalk for probing wounds.

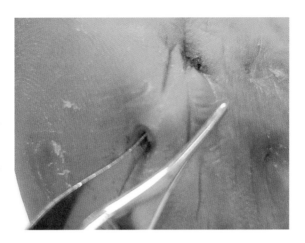

27A A neuropathic foot has developed colour change and blistering. This arises from an area of bleeding within callus. It is impossible to tell how extensive the problem is.
27B Debridement of the foot removes callus and de-roofs the blistered area, revealing extensive tissue damage and infection.

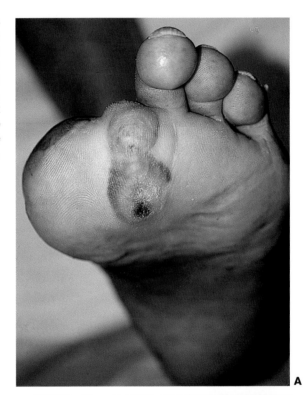

A

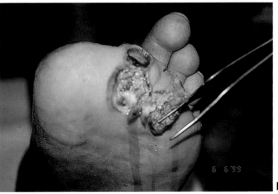

B

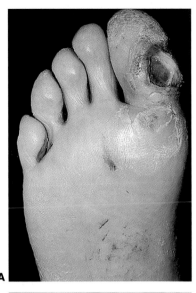

A

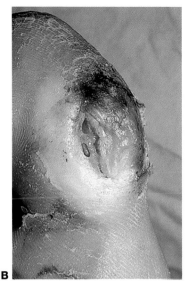

B

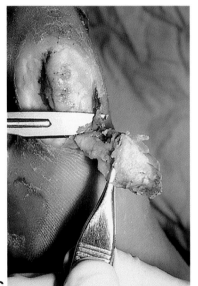

C

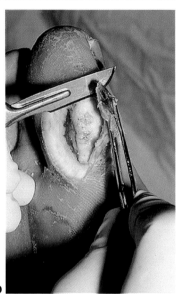

D

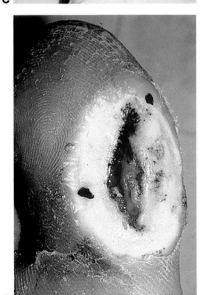

E

28A Neuropathic ulcer. The patient has developed a neuropathic ulcer on the medial plantar surface of the 1st toe, associated with overloading due to hallux rigidus.

28B A close-up view of the ulcer, revealing surrounding macerated callus. **28C** The podiatrist is removing callus using a "scalpel and forceps" technique where the callus is grasped with the forceps and gently pulled, thus applying tension, which makes it easier for the scalpel blade to cut through the material.

28D Callus is removed from the opposite edge of the ulcer.

28E The ulcer has been fully debrided.

29A Tannenbaumitis. This lady developed an unusual papular rash on both arms. The problem developed after she decorated a Christmas tree and sustained numerous needle-stick injuries. She decorated a Christmas tree every year and had never had a similar reaction; however, this tree was particularly expensive because it had been sprayed to prevent the needles dropping.

29B Close-up view of the lesions. The rash resolved on the fourth day of Christmas.

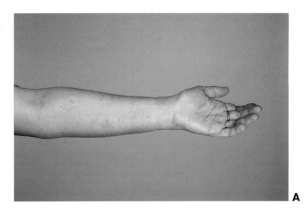

A

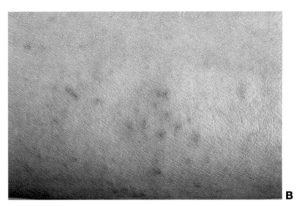

B

30 Rat bites. This picture is of a condition that is rarely seen in the United Kingdom, but is very common in developing countries. These are rat bites on the feet of a destitute man with alcoholic neuropathy who slept by a railway line that was infested with rats. His boots had holes in them and he was woken by the rats tugging at his feet, but only after they had already attacked and injured three toes.

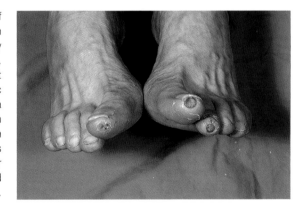

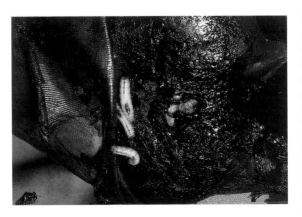

31 Wild maggots (traumatic myiasis). This elderly Afro-Caribbean patient was brought to the Foot Clinic by his daughter. She had visited him at home, noticed a curious odour and found a gangrenous foot infested with maggots. Blood glucose was 15mmol/L indicating a diagnosis of diabetes. He was admitted for intravenous antibiotics and surgical debridement. The foot could not be revascularised and was amputated: it was very ischaemic with extensive necrosis. The larvae were taken to the Microbiology department for identification; they were "flesh fly" larvae (Sarcophaga sp.).

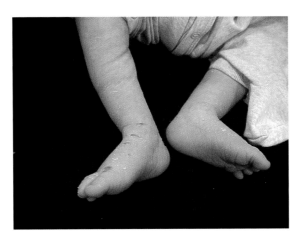

32 Infantile eczema. This baby has developed erythema, pruritis and fissuring of the feet and legs. He was referred to the Dermatology Department; the diagnosis was infantile eczema (atopic dermatitis). There was a history of atopy in the family; his father has eczema and asthma.

33A This is an early presenting partial thickness burn with blistering of the 3rd and 4th toes and lateral border of the foot.

33B Late presenting, full-thickness burns of the 1st toes of each foot from contact with a hot water pipe. The wound bed is necrotic.

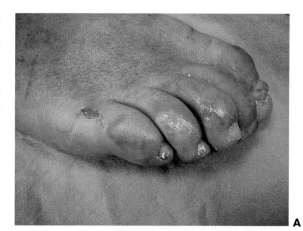

A

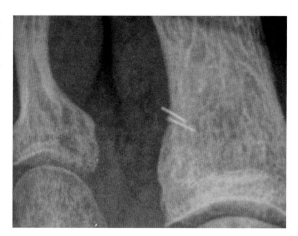

B

34 X-ray of foreign body; the patient was walking without shoes and trod on a staple gun, which fired two staples into the sole of his foot.

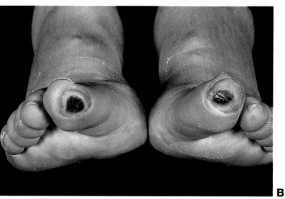

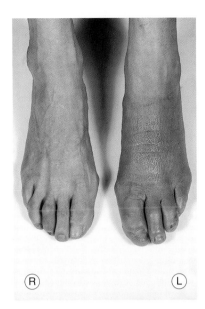

35 Dermatitis, cellulitis or Charcot's osteoarthropathy? This is contact dermatitis; the erythema has resulted from skin irritation caused by an occlusive bandage, around the left foot.

R   L

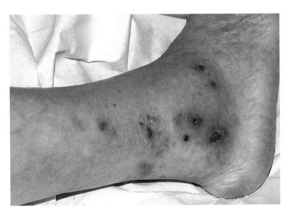

36 What is the cause of these palpable purpura? These lesions had central necrotic areas and biopsy showed a leucocytoclastic vasculitis.

37 Malignancy or blood within callus? Malignant lesions can sometimes be difficult to differentiate from callus with extravasation. It is important not to miss acral lentiginous melanomas, which are a specific presentation of cutaneous melanomas developing on the sole or toenail bed. If there is any doubt, patients should be referred to the Dermatology Department without delay.

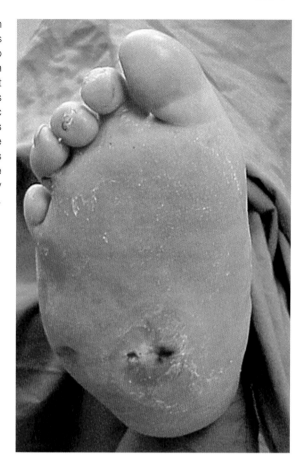

38 Tinea pedis infection or dermatitis? There is erythema and blistering particularly on the 2nd toe. This was contact dermatitis secondary to an over-the-counter cream. Tinea pedis is found more commonly between the toes and on the soles rather than on the dorsal surface of the foot.

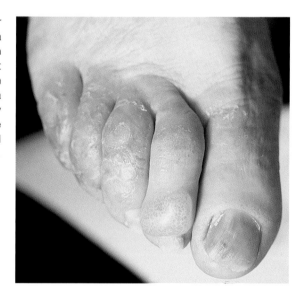

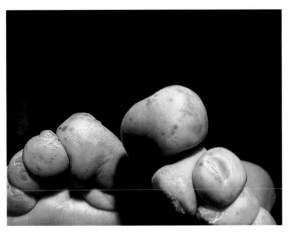

39 Vasculitis or micro-emboli? Multiple lesions indicating small infarctions in a patient with iliac atherosclerotic disease, from which showers of emboli escaped to the distal circulation.

Rheumatological disorders

Introduction

This chapter deals with rheumatological diseases, including rheumatoid arthritis, osteoarthritis, ankylosing spondilitis, scleroderma, Raynaud's syndrome, systemic lupus erythematosus, psoriasis and gout. We have included psoriasis in this chapter because some patients develop psoriatic arthropathy and in podiatric literature it is regarded as an inflammatory disease.

All of these conditions are painful and depressing for the patient and sometimes fail to respond well to treatment. Foot clinic patients with these problems will often be under the joint care of other departments: a podiatrist colleague of ours who ran a special weekly Foot Clinic for rheumatoid patients worked very closely with the Rheumatology Department.

Rheumatoid arthritis

1.1A Rheumatoid arthritis: dorsal view of the hands. This patient has had severe rheumatoid arthritis for many years. Her fingers are drifting laterally with ulnar deviation at the metacarpophalangeal joints. There are rheumatoid nodules at these joints and interphalangeal joints. **1.1B** Plantar view of the same hands.

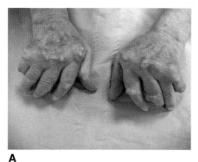
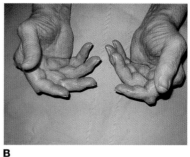

A   **B**

1.2 Bony changes in rheumatoid arthritis: erosion. This X-ray is of the foot of a 57-year-old woman with rheumatoid arthritis. There is severe hallux valgus deformity and an erosion of the heads of the 1st metatarsal and the 5th metatarsal. The sesamoids are displaced, and there is subluxation of the metatarsophalangeal joints.

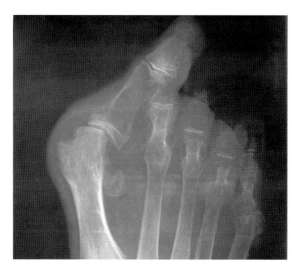

1.3 Rheumatoid foot. Callosities are present under very prominent metatarsal heads and distal displacement of the fibro-fatty cushions. When the patient first came to the foot clinic she wore court shoes and complained of severe pain on walking. The patient was issued with surgical shoes with deep wide toe boxes and cushioned insoles and was much more comfortable in them. She wore her new shoes whenever she was on her feet and the callus stopped forming. Our special weekly Foot Clinic for rheumatoid patients, run by Karen Larkin, a podiatrist who specialised in these disorders, meant that patients could be seen very frequently and had rapid emergency access if their feet became painful.

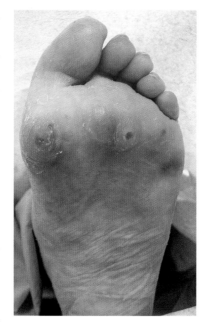

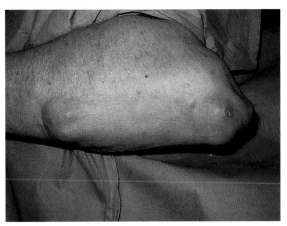

1.4 Rheumatoid nodules. These are present on the olecranon of the elbow and the extensor aspect of the forearm of a patient with rheumatoid arthritis. When these nodules are present on the feet they may lead to shoe-fitting problems. If rheumatoid nodules are subjected to pressure from shoes they may ulcerate and surgical excision may be the most practical solution.

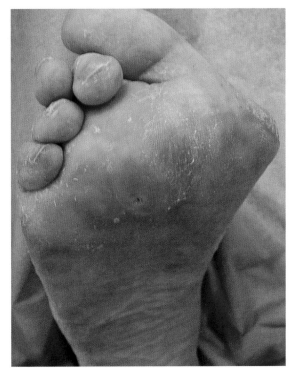

1.5 Hallux valgus deformity and ulcer in rheumatoid arthritis. There is severe hallux valgus deformity and the 3rd toe is dorsally displaced. The 3rd metatarsal head is prominent with overlying soft-tissue swelling and a small sinus has developed.

1.6 Rheumatoid arthritis with hallux valgus deformity. There is displacement of fibro-fatty padding, prominent 1st, 2nd and 3rd metatarsal heads with soft-tissue swelling, and small painful tissue breakdowns.

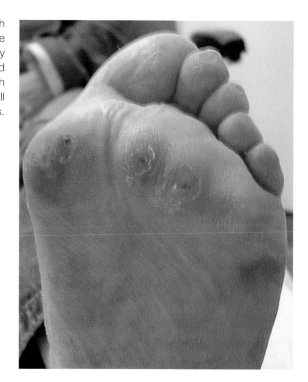

1.7A Ulcer on the heel of a patient with rheumatoid arthritis. This lady was obese, with a body mass index of 34, and the problem began when she walked barefoot and stepped on a drawing pin. She felt little pain from the injury or from the ulcer. **1.7B** The same foot after debridement. Callus has been removed from around the ulcer to reduce pressure, to ascertain the true dimensions of the wound and to allow it to drain. An ulcer swab showed no significant growth, and an X-ray showed no bony changes in the underlying calcaneum. The patient was advised to rest the foot, which healed in 3 months. Pain was reduced because of neuropathy, but was not absent. The patient used a wheelchair around the house and whenever she went out, until the ulcer healed. She could not use crutches because her wrists and elbows were painful when she did.

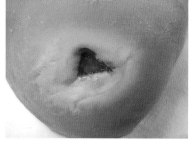

A

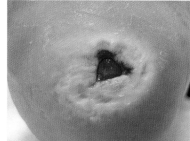

B

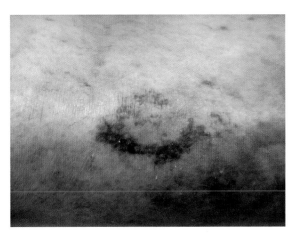

1.8 Purpura in rheumatoid arthritis. Non-blanching petechiae and eccymoses as a presentation of thrombocytopaenic purpura following gold salt therapy for rheumatoid arthritis. The purpura resolved spontaneously after cessation of the drug.

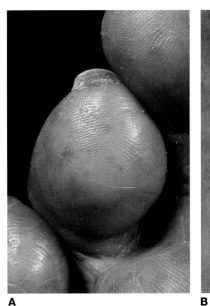

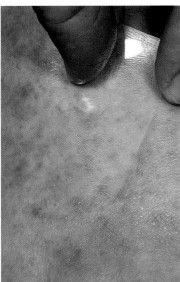

1.9A Vasculitic lesions in patient with rheumatoid arthritis. The patient has developed non-blanching lesions. Such vasculitic lesions are seen in patients with destructive rheumatoid arthritis associated with nodules and extra-articular complications.
1.9B Vasculitis. A piece of glass is being pressed against the skin to demonstrate the non-blanching nature of vasculitic lesions.

A　　　　　　　　　　**B**

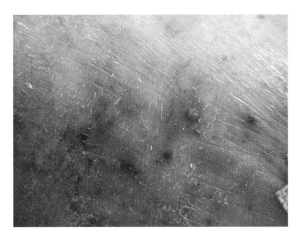

1.10 Secondary infection of vasculitic lesions: note the pustular appearance.

1.11 If infection in vasculitic lesions is not treated aggressively the results can be disastrous. This patient developed an extensive lower limb vasculitic rash of unknown cause, which was complicated by a polymicrobial infection.

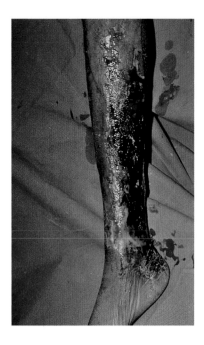

Osteoarthritis

1.12A Osteoarthritis and hallux rigidus. This patient used to play football in boots that were tight-fitting. He now has severe osteoarthritis with loss of joint space at the 1st metatarsal phalangeal joints, sclerotic joint margins, flattening of the 1st metatarsal head and lipping.

1.12B Some patients with hallux rigidus develop callus on the medial plantar aspect of the hallux, as seen in this patient.

1.12C Same patient after removal of callus from the plantar surface of the hallux.

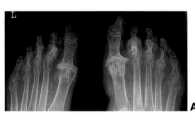

A

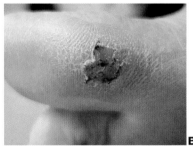

B

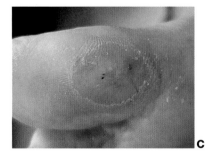

C

Ankylosing spondylitis

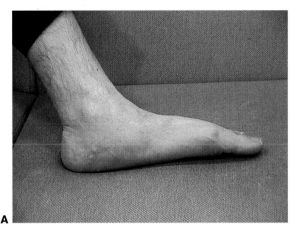

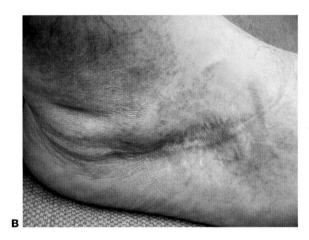

1.13A Ankylosing spondylitis. This 29-year-old man has ankylosing spondylitis, with pain and stiffness of his back, neck and shoulders on waking in the morning, and intermittent bouts of iritis and plantar fasciitis. He was born with grossly valgus feet and had bilateral Grise fusions aged 10. **1.13B** The other foot of same patient following triple arthrodesis at age 25. The brown staining is haemosiderin, which is frequently seen in areas that have undergone inflammation.

Scleroderma

1.14A Scleroderma. Scleroderma is a multisystem disorder with sclerotic, inflammatory and vascular abnormalities of skin and various internal organs. The feet of this patient with systemic sclerosis show blue discolouration, ulceration and early necrosis. This results from arteritis of the medium-sized arteries. The feet are very painful.

1.14B Close-up view of the left foot. The 1st toe is blue and pre-gangrenous. **1.14C** Plantar view of left foot. There is pallor and patchy purple discolouration.

1.14D Close-up view of 1st toe of right foot showing blue discolouration and necrosis.

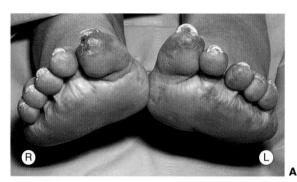

A

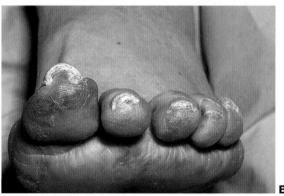

B

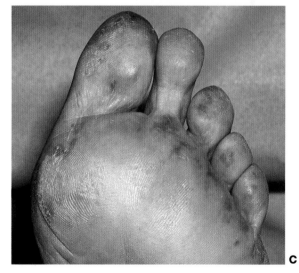

C

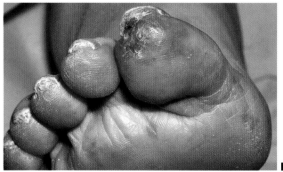

D

Raynaud's syndrome

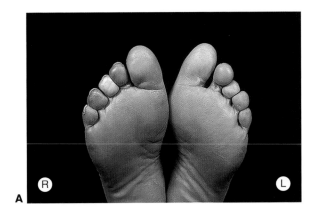

A

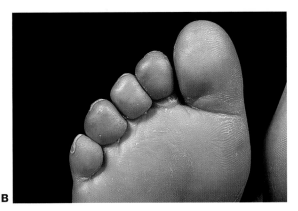

B

1.15A Raynaud's syndrome in a patient with CREST syndrome (**c**alcinosis, **R**aynaud's phenomenon, **e**sophagitis, **s**clerodactyly and **t**elangiectasia: the prognosis is less serious than for systemic sclerosis). This patient arrived at the clinic on a very cold day after standing in a bus queue waiting for a bus for several minutes. Her right 3rd toe is waxy white and the 2nd and 4th toes are very dusky.

1.15B The right foot after sitting in the warm clinic for 20 minutes. The whiteness is resolved and the toe has become pink again. The other toes are slightly dusky but have improved in the warmth of the Foot Clinic.

Systemic lupus erythematosus

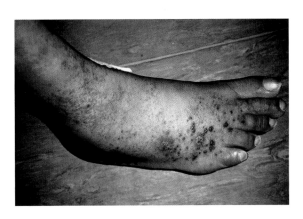

1.16 Systemic lupus erythematosus vasculitis. This lady developed systemic lupus in her twenties. These dark purpuric lesions result from vasculitis.

Psoriasis

1.17A Psoriatic legs. Note the variable degrees of erythema and scaling, and the island of normal tissue on the erythematous left shin. A frequent site for psoriatic plaques is the anterior shin of the lower leg. The right leg shows a common site of psoriasis on the anterior knee extending on to the lower leg. **1.17B** Close-up view of the left leg. **1.17C** Psoriatic hand. This patient has plaques of disease over the metacarpophalangeal joints, consisting of an erythematous papule with characteristic silver scales, typical of psoriasis vulgaris.

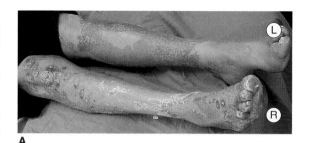

A

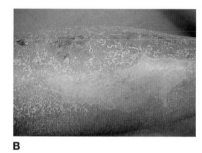

B

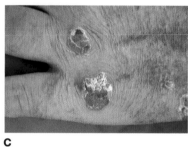

C

1.18A Psoriasis vulgaris on dorsum of foot. This elderly patient has psoriatic plaques consisting of red demarcated lesions and shiny white scales. The lesions come and go and are worst when he is under stress. When his feet are affected he wears socks and sandals to avoid shoe pressure on the plaques. **1.18B** Patch of psoriasis. This developed under a plaster cast and was at first thought to be a fungal infection.

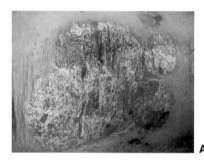

A

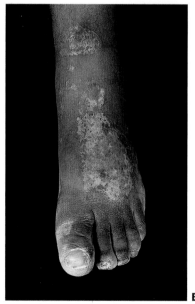

B

10

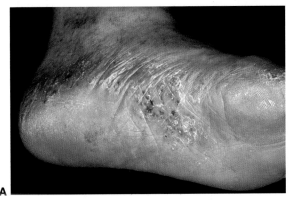

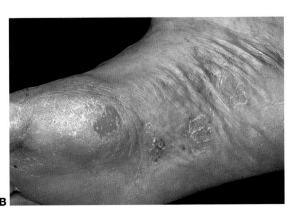

1.19A Pustular psoriasis. Lesions start as yellow pustules that do not rupture but dry up and become dark brown and scaly within a background of erythema. Pustular psoriasis is often mistaken for infected tinea pedis and also for contact dermatitis. Another differential diagnosis is Reiter's syndrome with keratoderma blennorrhagicum, which is characterized by psoriasiform lesions. **1.19B** Pustular psoriasis. Well demarcated, red and scaly plaques on the sole.

Gout

1.20A Gouty hands. The classical site for gout is the great hallux, but it may affect other parts of the body. In this patient the proximal interphalangeal joint of the 5th finger of the left hand and the distal interphalangeal joint of the 4th finger of the right hand are affected.

1.20B Close-up view of the left 5th finger showing inflammation and swelling of the proximal interphalangeal joint.

1.20C Close-up view of gout affecting distal interphalangeal joint of the 4th finger of the right hand. The whitish area is a gouty tophus, with deposits of uric acid crystals.

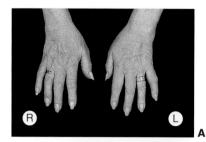

A

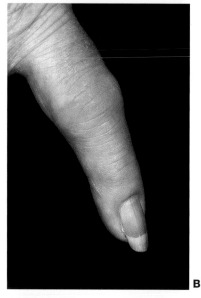

B

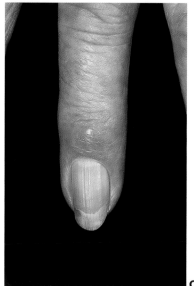

C

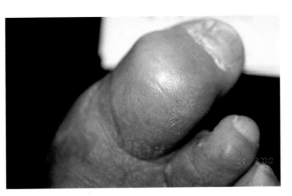

1.21 Acute gouty toe. This patient presented with agonizing pain, redness and swelling of the 1st toe. She was prescribed non-steroidal anti-inflammatory therapy until the acute episode had resolved and allopurinol was then prescribed to prevent relapse.

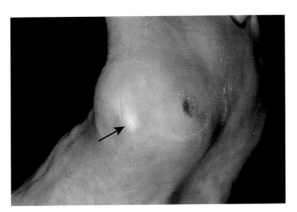

1.22 Gout in 1st metatarsophalangeal joint. This patient has diabetes, peripheral neuropathy and peripheral vascular disease. Following a successful distal bypass he had begun to develop plantar callus over the 1st metatarsal head, with a small breakdown. He then presented with a warm swelling over the 1st metatarsophalangeal joint with whitish discolouration (see arrow) on the medial surface that was diagnosed as a urate deposit.

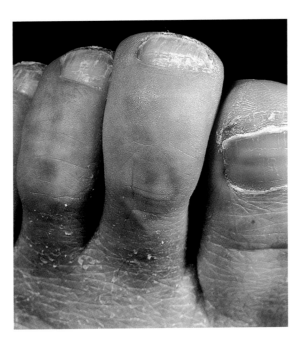

1.23 Gouty tophus on dorsum of 2nd toe. Sometimes these lesions ulcerate and exude whitish material. If the crystalline deposits within the tophus are carefully evacuated the area will usually heal.

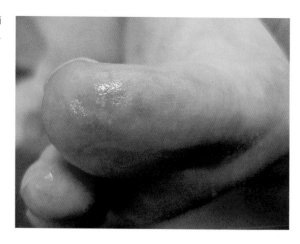

1.24 Several small gouty tophi are visible on this toe.

Infection

Introduction

Infection is a great destroyer of the foot. Many patients seen in the Foot Clinic with infections are immuno-compromised by virtue of concurrent health conditions. Infection is rarely a primary cause of foot ulceration, but frequently complicates breaks in the skin. Micro-organisms that are resistant to common antibiotics are more and more frequently encountered.

Infection is a major complication of the neuropathic foot and in particular in diabetes, although we have seen severe infection in patients with lower limb neuropathies from other causes. However, it is our impression that infection in these non-diabetic neuropathies is less frequently seen than in diabetic patients with neuropathy and runs a less devastating course.

It is essential to diagnose foot infection early, by carefully searching for early signs and symptoms, and to treat infection aggressively. Even a low-grade infection will delay or prevent healing, and spreading infection will cause wounds to deteriorate with alarming rapidity. The structure and function of the feet, and the fact that they are frequently covered by shoes and, therefore, are not observed closely, can make infection a serious problem.

This chapter shows examples of soft-tissue infection, osteomyelitis and fungal infections affecting the feet and legs. Unless mentioned otherwise, these infections have developed in diabetic patients.

Soft-tissue infections

2.1 Cellulitis in an Afro-Caribbean foot. The left foot and leg are infected. Cellulitis is less evident in a pigmented foot. The two feet should always be carefully compared. In this case, the right, unaffected, leg and foot are much paler.

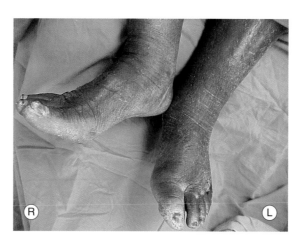

2.2 Peripheral cyanosis as a sign of infection. These infected feet show marked erythema indicative of cellulitis with cyanosis in the distal areas because of a failure to meet the increased oxygen demands of the infected peripheral tissues.

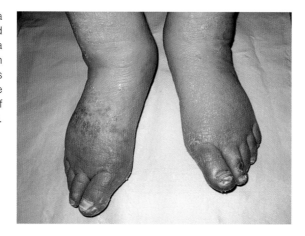

2.3 Mild cellulitis. The 2nd toe is a little pink. The portal of entry was a crack between the toes.

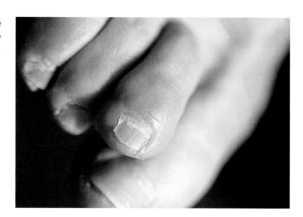

CHAPTER 2 Infection

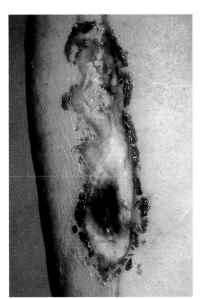

2.4 Slough and necrosis in leg wound. A moist, infected distal bypass wound is complicated by slough and necrosis. This can be difficult to sharp debride because it is not easy to grasp with forceps, but it can be dried with gauze so that it will be more straightforward to grasp and cut away.

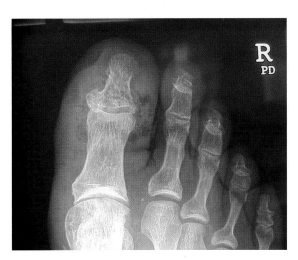

2.5 Gas in tissues. This patient attended as an emergency with brawny swelling of the 1st toe. He felt unwell, with fever and rigors. Palpation of the 1st toe revealed crepitus, and gas in the soft tissues was evident on X-ray. This is a clinical emergency; if the infecting organism producing the gas is clostridium perfringens then gas gangrene and death can ensue. This patient was admitted for intravenous antibiotics and surgical debridement. The gas-producing organisms were Bacteroides and Escherichia coli.

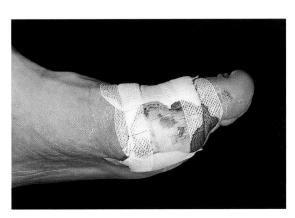

2.6 Strike-through. Strike-through occurs when a dressing has absorbed so much exudate that it shows through on the opposite side to the wound interface. Increased amounts of exudate produced by a wound and any exudates that are not clear and serous, or are malodorous, are important signs of infection.

2.7A Pseudomonas aeruginosa infection. A dressing is removed from a varicose ulcer to reveal blue–green staining typical of infection with Pseudomonas aeruginosa. **2.7B** Infected 4th toe: part of the ulcer bed is stained green indicating Pseudomonas infection. There is often a characteristic fusty, musty, mousy odour associated with this organism.

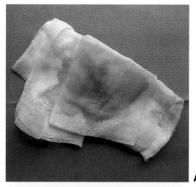

A

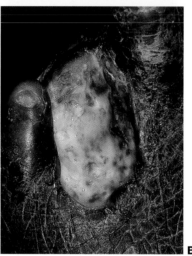

B

2.8A Tracking. Tracking of pus under callus is an important warning sign of infection. This patient has neuropathy and neglected callus. Pressure from the callus has led to tissue necrosis and ulceration of the soft tissues beneath the callus. Because the overlying callus is intact, the ulcer cannot drain. Pus is tracking under the callus. **2.8B** The foot after debridement to reveal the ulcer and cavity of tracking pus, which has been drained.

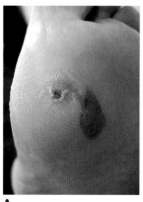

A

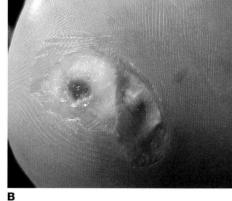

B

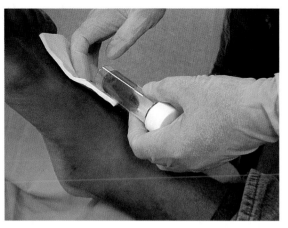

2.9 Pus from infected foot. This Afro-Caribbean patient had a severely cellulitic foot. The tube contains blood-stained pus drained from the foot, which was sent to the laboratory for microscopy and culture. Whenever possible, sending specimens of pus or tissue is preferable to sending a swab; the harvest of micro-organisms is likely to be better.

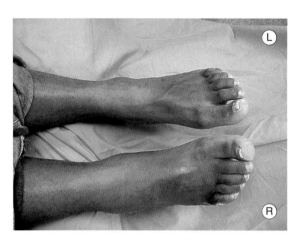

2.10 Comparing feet. It is always very important to check both feet. In this case, the right foot is infected. Compared with the left foot, the right foot is warm and swollen. The patient was Afro-Caribbean so colour change is not as obvious as it would be in a Caucasian. There was a small wound on the 5th toe of the right foot.

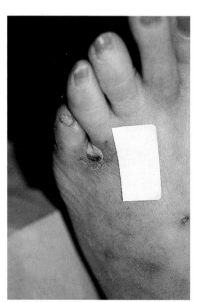

2.11 Dressings can mask an infection. This patient had a painful crack in the web space between the 4th and 5th toes and applied an occlusive dressing. This masked the foot and she could not see that the problem was deteriorating, although she was aware that the pain level was not decreasing. After 1 week she removed the occlusive dressing and revealed a sloughy, necrotic area in the web space. The wound grew a combination of Staphylococcus aureus and beta-haemolytic Streptococcus group B.

2.12 Neglected abrasion. This elderly lady caught her leg on the step of an ambulance when leaving the hospital after a visit to the Foot Clinic. She did not tell the ambulance staff, nor seek treatment, as she thought the abrasion was too superficial to make a fuss. This photograph was taken 3 weeks later, by which time the wound was much larger and sloughy, with associated cellulitis.

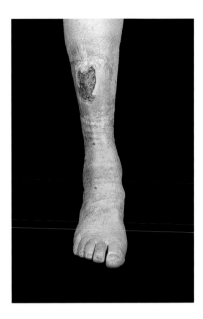

2.13 Colour change in wound bed. A deep, infected neuropathic ulcer. The wound bed, formerly a healthy pink granulating bed, is greyish and a discharge is running out of the ulcer.

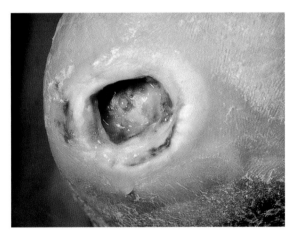

2.14 Cellulitis. The 2nd toe is infected. The portal of entry was a blister caused by a shoe rub. Cellulitis is spreading up the foot, and the patient was admitted and given intravenous antibiotics.

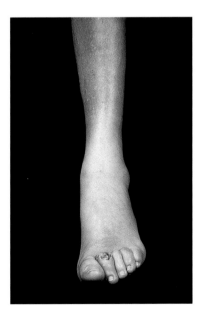

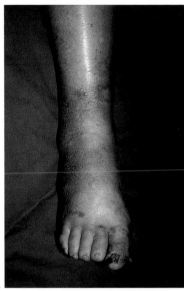

A

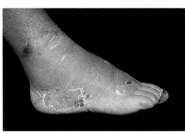

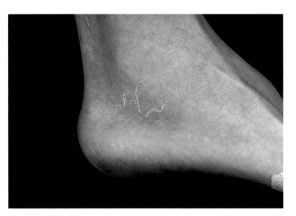

B

2.15A Toxic shock and septicaemia. This non-diabetic patient with a chronic in-growing toenail underwent partial nail avulsion with phenolysation of the nail matrix. She was apparently otherwise in good health. Within 16 hours she developed pain in her thigh followed by swelling of the limb and feelings of malaise, nausea, tiredness and shivering. Her husband brought her to the Foot Clinic and had to carry her in as she could not walk. She was shocked, pyrexial and hypovolaemic and was immediately taken to Casualty, resuscitated, admitted and given intravenous antibiotics. Her progress was slow. A blood culture grew beta-haemolytic Streptococcus group A. She was discharged after 3 weeks.

2.15B The patient on the day of discharge. Note the extensive desquamation, which is common after a Streptococcal infection.

2.16 Post-infective desquamation. This patient had a small infected blister below his lateral malleolus. A swab grew Staphylococcus aureus and beta-haemolytic Streptococcus group B. After the wound healed there was desquamation of the previously cellulitic area.

2.17A Trauma and cellulitis leading to post-inflammatory hyperpigmentation. This shows anterior view of leg. This patient, aged 38 years, sustained an injury from an airport trolley on his posterior lower leg and developed severe cellulitis requiring hospital admission. The leg healed but there was post-inflammatory hyperpigmentation of the previously cellulitic area. **2.17B** Posterior view of the lower leg.

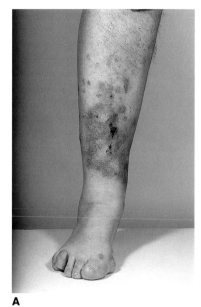

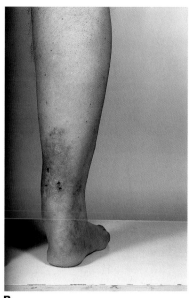

A

B

2.18A Blanching. This severely infected foot shows sub-ungual ulceration, bluish discolouration of the ulcerated 1st toe, and blanching of the lesser toes. Unless the infection is rapidly controlled, gangrene will supervene with alarming rapidity. **2.18B** A close-up view of the foot shows the sloughy ulcerated nail bed, and the blue discolouration, which is an early sign of septic vasculitis affecting the digital arteries.

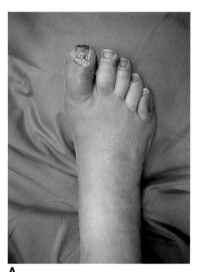

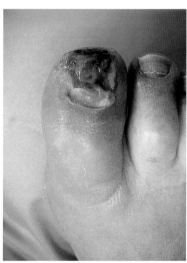

A

B

2.19 Septic vasculitis. The toes are becoming gangrenous. This is due to septic vasculitis. The portal of entry for infection was an ulcer on the plantar surface.

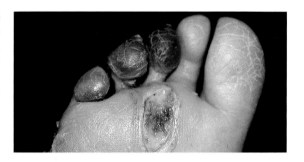

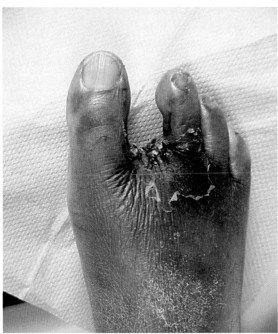 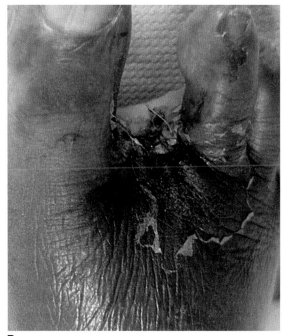

A **B**

2.20A Toe amputation. This patient has undergone amputation of his 2nd toe for wet necrosis. Swabs grew Staphylococcus aureus and beta-haemolytic Streptococcus group C. A strongly pigmented Afro-Caribbean skin can mask cellulitis, but a reddish tawny discolouration, skin wrinkles where oedema has resolved, and desquamation (often associated with a resolving Streptococcal infection) are apparent.

2.20B The same foot 4 days later. There is post-inflammatory hyperpigmentation. The wound was sutured, which is unwise in cases of severe infection.

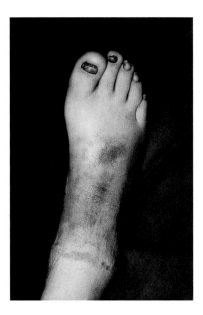

2.21 Severe infection in a diabetic foot. This patient presented at Casualty with a red, swollen foot. He was admitted and given intravenous antibiotics.

2.22 Severe infection with septic vasculitis. Septic vasculitis with septic thrombus occluding the digital arteries has led to gangrene of the 4th and 5th toes. Gangrene is extending onto the dorsum of the foot, and the 2nd and 3rd toes are pre-gangrenous. The pedal pulses were strong and bounding, and the patient had a diabetic peripheral neuropathy. Intravenous antibiotics and surgical removal of gangrenous tissues will save the leg and most of the foot. If the problem is detected when the toes first turn blue they can often be saved with antibiotic therapy.

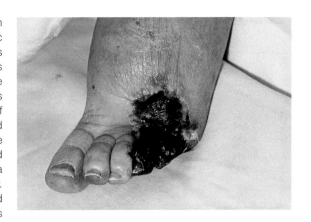

2.23 Drainage and debridement. This patient with diabetic retinopathy and neuropathy lived alone and was socially isolated. He had previously had lesser toe amputations. He presented very late at Casualty. He felt no pain in his foot and could not see the problem. He only sought help because he and his pet dog could smell "something terrible" and the dog was very restless and disturbed, and kept sniffing the foot and barking. Infection was tracking along the sole of the foot. He underwent extensive surgical debridement and drainage. Antibiotics alone are not adequate treatment for an infection of this severity.

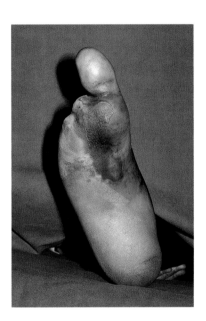

2.24 Traumatic leg ulcer with secondary infection. This ulcer commenced as an abrasion, which became infected with Staphylococcus aureus.

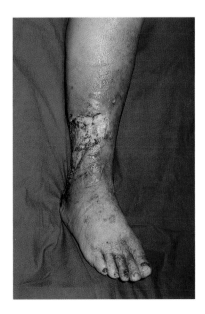

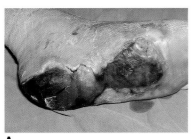 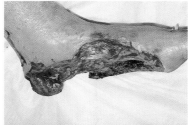

A **B**

2.25A Infective necrosis of heel and sole. This diabetic patient was in renal failure. There was a polymicrobial infection of Escherichia coli and Staphylococus aureus.
2.25B Same foot after debridement. This shows the extent of the necrosis.

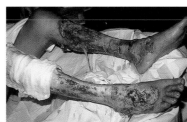

A

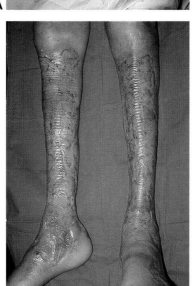

B

2.26A Vibrio vulnificus infection. This patient with cirrhosis of the liver went on holiday to Florida and ate raw oysters. He was not aware that some oysters are transported in un-refrigerated vans and may contain the micro-organism Vibrio vulnificus, a cholera-like organism that can cause gastro-intestinal problems and vasculitis. Within a few hours he was taken to the local emergency room, with diarrhoea, fever and hypotension. There is a primary enteritis complicated by a bacteraemia and then dissemination to the skin.
2.26B He was treated with tetracycline and split skin grafts and made a good recovery.

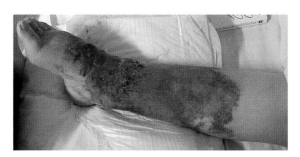

2.27 Pasteurella multocida. This lady with lymphoedema developed a small blister on the back of her ankle and allowed her small puppy to lick it. She developed redness, pain and throbbing, and deteriorated with alarming rapidity. A specimen grew pasteurella multocida, which is an organism commonly present in the saliva of cats and dogs. She was admitted to hospital and given intravenous amoxicillin/clavulanic acid. Pets should not be allowed to interfere with open wounds.

2.28 Post-infective desquamation. This patient presented with severe cellulitis of both feet and legs and was admitted for systemic antibiotics. Swabs grew a beta-haemolytic Streptococcus group B. He developed desquamation of large areas of skin on both feet, which is commonly seen after a Streptococcal infection. In the days of scarlet fever (systemic Streptococcal infection) it was common for patients to lose skin over their palms and soles.

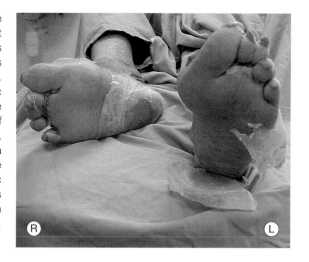

2.29A Varicose ulceration complicated by infection. This 80-year-old, non-diabetic lady had varicose veins and suffered from venous leg ulceration for many years. The ulceration also extended onto the dorsum of the foot. She was under the care of the community nurses and was referred to the hospital after the ulcers became infected. Rarity of infection of venous ulcers leading to gangrene probably explains the better outcome of venous leg ulcers compared to diabetic foot ulcers.
2.29B A view of the ulcer on the lateral ankle. **2.29C** A view of the dorsum of the foot, showing exposure of extensor tendons in the ulcer. **2.29D** A close-up view of extensor tendons laid bare by infection.

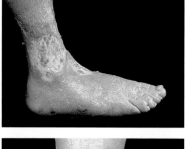

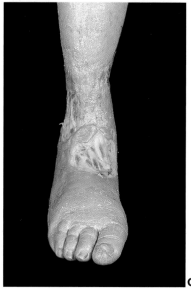

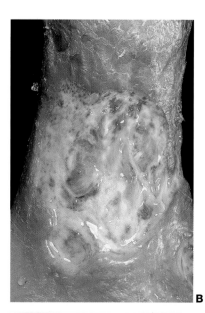

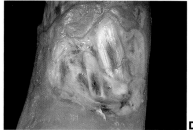

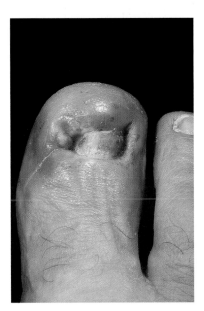

2.30 Partial nail avulsion complicated by infection. Note the greyish, macerated wound bed; this may be hard to differentiate from greyness and maceration caused by topical application of phenol to ablate the nail bed.

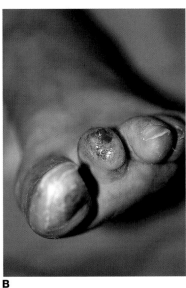

2.31 Plantar ulceration complicated by infection and wet necrosis. Note the necrotic areas in the wound bed and the surrounding cellulitis. There was a foul odour that drove the patient to seek help, and the debridings obtained at surgery grew Bacteroides, Pseudomonas aeruginosa and Staphylococcus aureus. Severe infections are frequently polymicrobial.

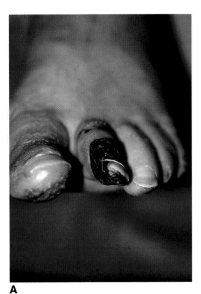 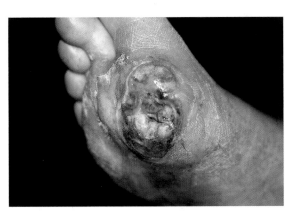

A **B**

2.32A Dry gangrene. This rare picture shows dry gangrene in a diabetic neuropathic foot with bounding pulses. The patient inadvertently cut his toe when performing nail care and the cut became infected. When the distal portion of the toe turned dusky blue, he visited his general practitioner who prescribed antibiotics. These controlled the infection and rendered the necrosis dry.

2.32B The same foot after the podiatrist has removed the gangrenous portion of the toe as an out patient procedure in the Foot Clinic. No local anaesthetic was required due to the neuropathy, and the foot was fully healed in 1 week.

2.33 Infected burn. This patient spilled boiling water on his neuropathic foot but did not seek help until his diabetic control became poor. The foot was infected and the larger blister covers a full-thickness burn.

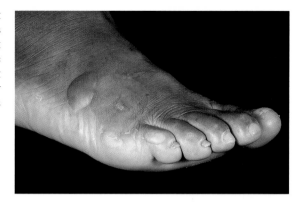

2.34 Infected pressure ulcer. This Afro-Caribbean patient was admitted to hospital after a stroke and developed sacral and heel pressure lesions. His left heel is now badly infected and has developed wet necrosis.

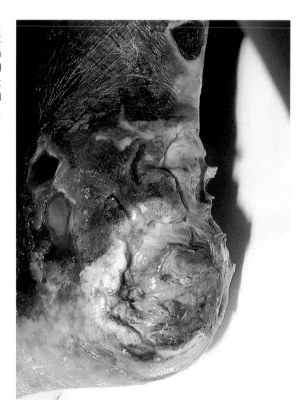

2.35A Infection, cellulitis and necrosis. The problem began with an interdigital crack from a fungal infection. The patient was a 62-year-old, socially isolated man. **2.35B** Close-up view of the foot.

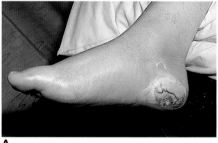

A

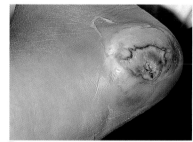

B

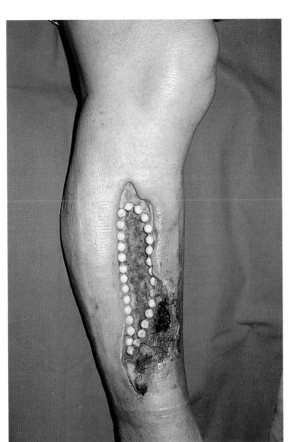

2.36 Infected wound treated with gentamicin beads. This diabetic ischaemic patient underwent a distal bypass and the leg wound became infected. Gentamicin impregnated beads were placed in the wound.

2.37 Infected trauma. This patient was walking barefoot and dropped a frozen chicken onto his foot causing an open wound. He applied a band aid. He developed swelling 3 days later and pain of the foot. He attended Casualty and was referred to the Foot Clinic. He was not known to be diabetic, but had a blood glucose of 15 mmol/L and a glycated haemoglobin of 11%. His pedal pulses were bounding. Diabetes and peripheral neuropathy were diagnosed. He was given antibiotics. A swab grew Staphylococcus aureus and flucloxacillin was prescribed. He was educated in foot care and attended the Foot Clinic regularly. He healed in 3 weeks and did not relapse. The outcome for dorsal wounds in the neuropathic foot is usually better than for wounds on plantar, weight-bearing sites, which are very prone to develop into indolent neuropathic ulcers.

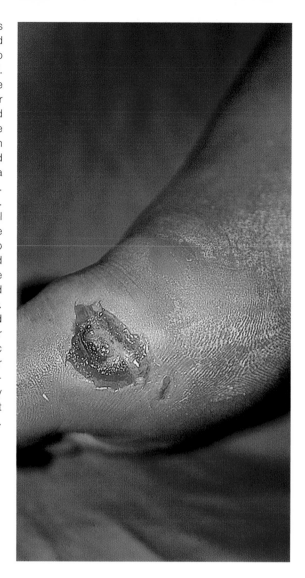

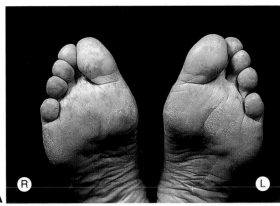

2.38A Rash from antibiotic sensitivity. The patient had an infected ischaemic ulcer and was given amoxicillin, flucloxacillin and metronidazole. He developed an itchy macular rash over his entire body probably due to penicillin allergy. **2.38B** Right foot of same patient. **2.38C** Close-up of same patient.

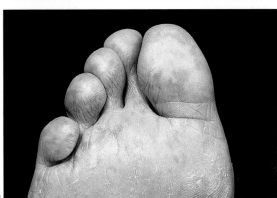

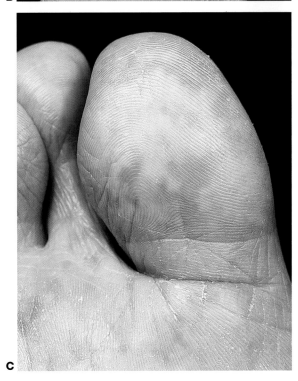

2.39A This patient presented with an infected ulcer on the medial aspect of the first metatarsal head. **2.39B** There was associated erythema on the dorsum of the foot. **2.39C** Cellulitis had spread to the lower leg. **2.39D** Close-up view of the infected ulcer. **2.39E** The patient was treated with amoxicillin, fludoxacillin and metronidazole and seen 1 week later when the infection was resolving, but the patient had developed a macular rash suggestive of an antibiotic allergy. **2.39F** A close-up view of the rash. It resolved after the antibiotics were discontinued, but during this period the foot was checked on a daily basis to detect any deterioration quickly.

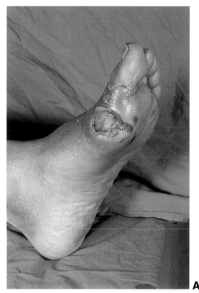

A

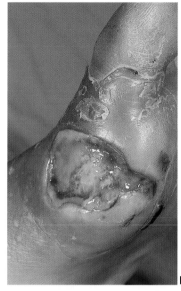

D

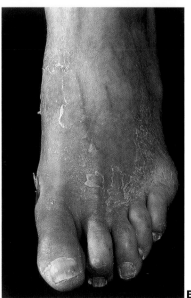

B

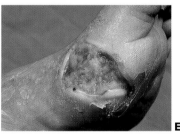

E

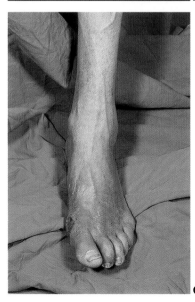

C

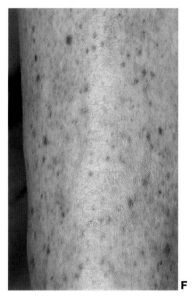

F

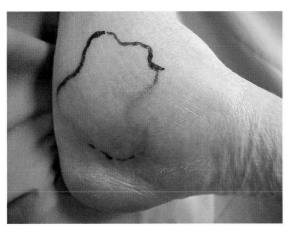

2.40 Differential diagnosis: is it infection or a Charcot ankle? The ankle was red, warm and swollen; the problem had arisen over the previous 2 days. X-ray showed no abnormality. On presentation, an ink tracing was made on the skin around the area of redness; within 24 hours it had extended beyond the lower part of the traced area, as shown, indicating a spreading infection. She was admitted for intravenous antibiotics.

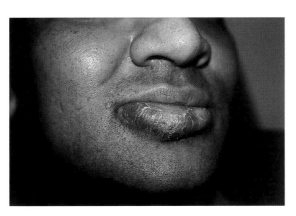

2.41 It is not only the feet that should be inspected. This patient had an abscess of the lip that was detected in the Foot Clinic at a routine appointment, and drained as an outpatient procedure in Accident and Emergency.

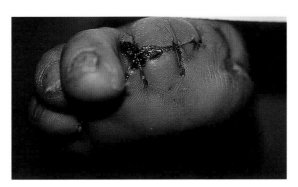

2.42 Dangers of suturing an infected foot. This patient underwent amputation of the 1st toe and 2nd toe for osteomyelitis. The surgeon undertook primary closure and sutured the wound. The foot was cellulitic 3 days later. The sutures were removed, revealing necrotic tissue and the patient needed a Lisfranc amputation.

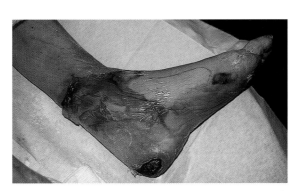

2.43 Overwhelming infection. This diabetic patient with neuropathy and end-stage renal failure, who was on haemodialysis, had a long history of forefoot ulcers and previous amputation of the 1st toe. He was admitted to his local hospital and developed an ulcer on his right heel. Within 1 week, he developed fulminating infection of the foot and ankle, and was seen in the Diabetic Foot Clinic. At surgery there was deep wet necrosis, gas in the tissues and total destruction of the ankle joint. He underwent major amputation.

Osteomyelitis

2.44 Bone infection. Sausage toe – a marker for osteomyelitis. Note also the shiny "pouting" convex surface of the associated ulcer. These signs are frequently associated with the presence of a sinus, through which it is possible to pass a probe right to the underlying bone or joint.

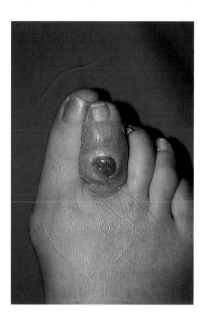

2.45 Sausage toe. This lady has a "sausage toe" (fusiform swelling and erythema of a toe), which is a marker for osteomyelitis. The dorsal ulcer looks small, clean and trivial, but probed to bone. The patient had dropped a heavy object on her foot 2 months previously. The 3rd toe nail had a subungual haematoma and the 2nd toe received a laceration on the dorsum. The patient applied a sticking plaster and did not seek treatment. Over the next few weeks she noticed a little discharge and the 2nd toe was throbbing. It then developed redness and fusiform swelling, at which point she came to the Foot Clinic via her general practitioner. X-ray revealed osteomyelitis. A sterile probe was inserted into the dorsal lesion and bone was touched; probing to bone is also diagnostic of osteomyelitis. The toe healed after a 3-month course of rifampicin and fucidin.

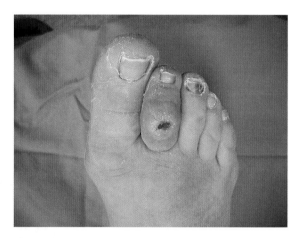

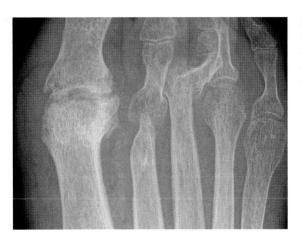

2.46 X-ray showing "sucked candy" appearance of the 2nd metatarsal. This is usually associated with chronic sepsis in a neuropathic ulcer.

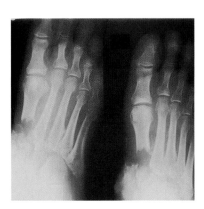

2.47 Osteomyelitis. This patient previously underwent amputation of the 4th and 5th toes and debridement of the 1st metatarsal for severe infection. The wound from the 1st metatarsal debridement never healed. X-ray (oblique and straight views) reveals osteomyelitis with fluffy appearance and crumbling of bone affecting the base of the 1st metatarsal.

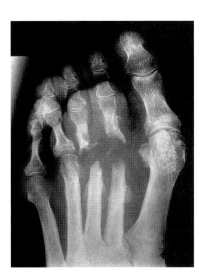

2.48 Osteomyelitis. This X-ray is of the foot of a 53-year-old, type 1 diabetic with neuropathic ulceration and reveals destruction of the 2nd and 3rd metatarsal heads by infection. No surgery had been performed on the foot.

2.49A Osteomyelitis. This patient with diabetic neuropathy had redness, pain, warmth and swelling of the right 1st toe. The differential diagnosis included infection, gout and Charcot's osteoarthropathy.

2.49B Straight and oblique-view X-rays. These revealed osteomyelitis with fragmentation of the distal area of the proximal phalanx. The patient had normal liver function and was treated for 3 months with oral fucidin and rifampicin, both of which are antibiotics with good bony penetration, and the bony changes resolved.

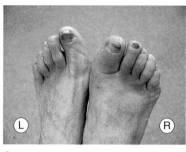
A

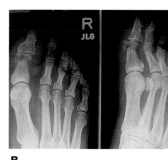
B

Fungal infections

2.50 Vesicular tinea. The vesicular rash on this patient's foot is due to infection with a fungus (tinea pedis). It was easily treated with topical terbinafine (Lamisil) 1% cream, applied once daily. Treatment was continued for 2 weeks after final resolution of symptoms to avoid re-infection.

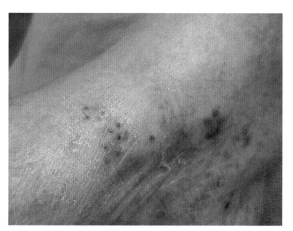

2.51 Vesicular tinea. Tinea pedis can present in different ways. This patient has had a vesicular rash, with associated erythema and desquamation. It was treated with topical canesten (clotrimazole 1% in isopropyl alcohol) spray and resolved within 2 weeks. The spray formulation is particularly useful when the interdigital area is affected.

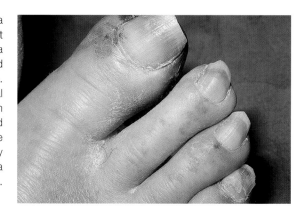

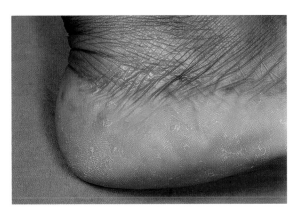

2.52 Moccasin tinea. This is tinea pedis in a moccasin distribution, with dry skin and vesicles.

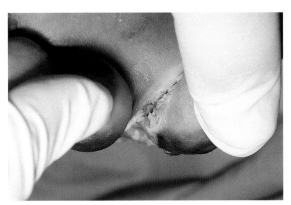

2.53 Interdigital tinea pedis. There is white maceration and erosion of the skin. This non-diabetic patient sought help because the foot smelled bad.

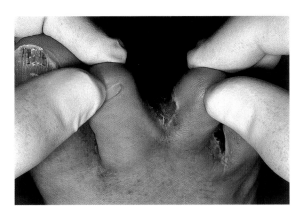

2.54 Interdigital erosion of tinea pedis. The nail of the 1st toe has onychomycosis.

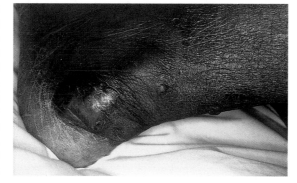

2.55 Plectophomella chromomycosis. This patient was a 52-year-old, Afro-Caribbean patient who was born and raised in Jamaica and came to the UK at the age of 30. The last time he had revisited Jamaica (or any tropical country) had been 17 years previous to this photograph being taken. He had developed leg ulcers 6 months previously, which were assumed to be varicose and treated by the community nurses. When he was referred to the Foot Clinic we also noted the presence of macules on his feet and legs, some of which had central sinuses, which were draining dark oily fluid. Some of this material was expressed and sent for microscopy and culture. It contained fungal hyphae, and a deep fungal infection – chromomycosis – was diagnosed. This is extremely rarely seen in temperate climates.

The patient was diabetic, and also pre-leukaemic and severely immunosuppressed. In these circumstances, unusual infections are sometimes seen.

The infecting organism was Plectophomella, a fungus usually seen in elm trees; the patient had worked as a carpenter.

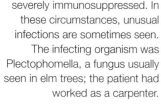

Circulatory disorders

Introduction

Ischaemia is the most common cause of major amputation in the United Kingdom. It is essential to detect ischaemia early and to follow patients carefully. Regular palpation of pedal pulses and inspections for early warning signs of ischaemia are both important aspects of monitoring ischaemic patients. A small hand-held Doppler is an essential piece of equipment for a Foot Clinic, and a machine for measuring oxygen tension in the skin (transcutaneous oxymetry) is an expensive piece of equipment, but very useful. Collaboration with a fully equipped vascular laboratory is useful. The vascular surgeons and interventional radiologists are important members of the multidisciplinary Foot Clinic team: at King's, the Foot Clinic team has joint weekly clinics and a weekly interventional radiology meeting.

Modern techniques for improving perfusion, including percutaneous transluminal balloon angioplasty (often offered as a day-case procedure) and arterial bypass are very effective, but patients who undergo these procedures should be followed long-term in the Foot Clinic and regularly reassessed. "Once ischaemic, always high-risk" is an important maxim. This chapter shows examples of: acute ischaemia, when there has been a sudden occlusion of a major artery in the leg within the previous 24 hours; critical ischaemia, when the perfusion of the lower limb is severely limited, resulting in the foot becoming extensively necrotic if the condition is not improved, and chronic ischaemia, when there is a severe but stable reduction of perfusion to the lower limb.

It also shows examples of tissue necrosis and emboli in the ischaemic foot. Other circulatory conditions demonstrated are venous disease, lymphoedema and chilblains (perniosis). Finally, revascularization of the ischaemic limb is considered.

Acute ischaemia

3.1 Acute ischaemia. This diabetic patient presented as an emergency with pain and numbness of recent duration in the foot and lower leg, which was cold, mottled and pulseless. There was a clear demarcation line from a warm, well-perfused leg at mid calf level to a cold lower limb. Doppler studies revealed no detectable flow in the foot. The patient was admitted immediately under the vascular team and underwent distal bypass. The foot was salvaged.

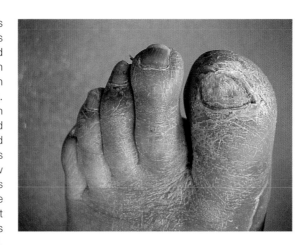

3.2 Acute ischaemia. This patient developed pallor, mottling and paraesthesiae in the foot, with severe weakness. He was admitted the same day and underwent arterial bypass, which saved the leg.

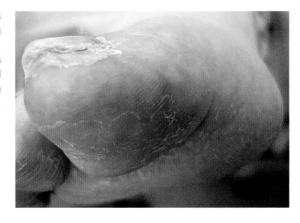

Critical ischaemia

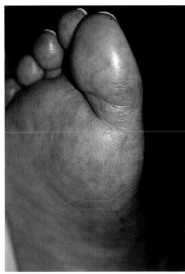

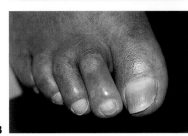

3.3A Critical ischaemia. This foot is cold, with impalpable pulses and there is severe rest pain. **3.3B** Pale nail beds. Note the pale nail beds, which can be a sign of severe ischaemia.

A

B

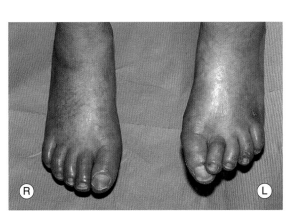

3.4 Pink painful cold ischaemic feet. Feet showing exaggerated hyperaemia on dependency after initial limb elevation.

3.5 Sock marks. The cold, pink, pulseless ischaemic foot is very vulnerable to trauma. This patient has been wearing socks that are too tight and have marked the skin. A change to more suitable hose is urgently required; overly tight socks and prominent seams can cause ulceration in the ischaemic foot. Indeed, the right foot shows a red mark – pre-ulcerative – caused by pressure from the tight sock.

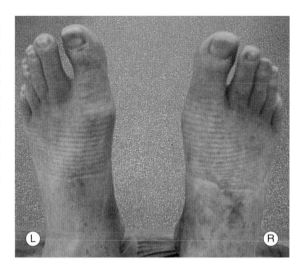

3.6 Ischaemic ulcer. This is a very painful ulcer in a characteristic site over a bony metatarsal prominence. The surrounding skin is cyanotic.

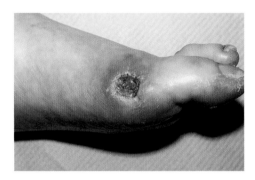

3.7 Critical ischaemia. This is a cold, pulseless, dusky, ischaemic foot in a diabetic patient on dialysis. There is a small ulcer on the medial plantar aspect of the 1st toe.

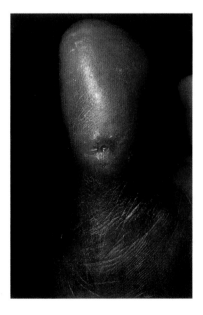

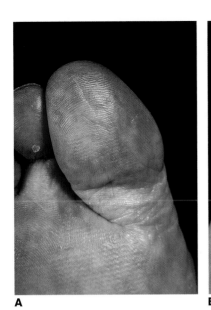

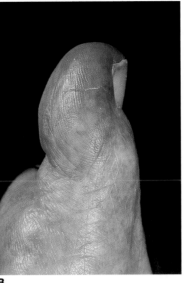

A   **B**

3.8A Critical ischaemia: the 1st toe is bluish and mottled. **3.8B** Lateral view of the same toe.

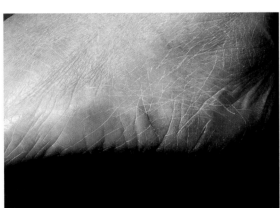

3.9 Incipient ischaemic ulceration. This diabetic ischaemic patient has very dry, fragile skin around the heels. The skin is cracking, and each fissure has a rim of erythema. Ulceration is incipient and the foot is so ischaemic that any ulcers are unlikely to heal unless vascular intervention is feasible.

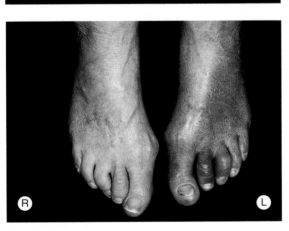

3.10 Critically ischaemic foot. Compare the ischaemic left foot with the right foot. The left foot is dusky, cold, pulseless and painful.

3.11 A pair of critically ischaemic feet. Thin, shiny, atrophic, cyanosed skin in a patient with critical ischaemia.

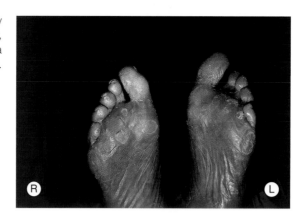

3.12A Local positional ischaemia. This lady has a pink, icy cold, pulseless ischaemic foot with a sloughy ulcer in a classical site on the lateral border of the foot. In such patients, ulceration involving the lateral malleolus is also common. In this picture, a white ischaemic patch is apparent over the lateral malleolus. (The patient is extending the toes). **3.12B** The same patient. When she flexes her toes, the white ischaemic area regains its colour.

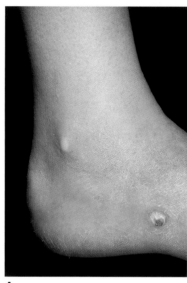

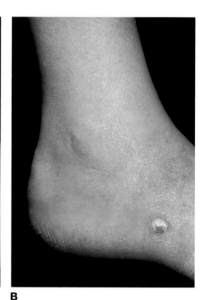

A   B

Chronic ischaemia

3.13 Chronic ischaemia and ulceration. This diabetic patient with chronic ulceration of the nail bed of the 3rd toe had ischaemia with an ankle brachial pressure index of 0.52. She was seen every fortnight at the Foot Clinic, but presented as an emergency complaining of increased pain and weakness of the foot and leg. Doppler studies revealed a pressure index of 0.22. She underwent angioplasty, following which the pressure index rose to 0.71 and the ulcer healed in 5 months.

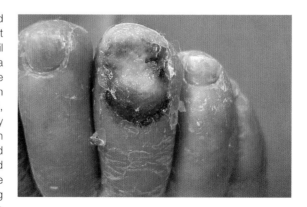

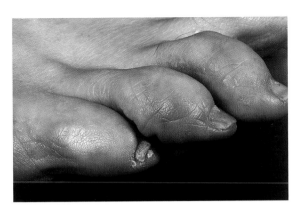

3.14 A red mark – the precursor of an ischaemic ulcer. This diabetic patient with peripheral vascular disease has developed red marks on the lateral border of the 3rd, 4th and 5th toes from a tight shoe. The patient will rapidly develop an ischaemic ulcer unless the pressure is reduced. Patients with a problem caused by the shoe should not leave the clinic wearing the same shoe; the footwear needs to be adjusted or replaced.

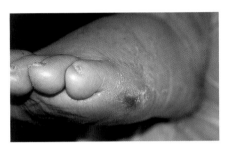

3.15 Oedema in the ischaemic foot. Swelling has rendered the shoe too tight. Resulting pressure on the margins of the foot has led to a pressure point on the lateral border, with an erythematous area and incipient ulceration.

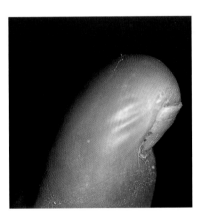

3.16 Early sign of ischaemic ulcer. Early ischaemic ulcer presenting as a blistered area of discolouration on the 1st toe of a diabetic patient.

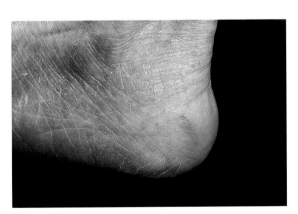

3.17 Early shoe rub. This ischaemic foot is being subjected to rubbing from the shoe. Unless this is addressed urgently it will cause an ulcer.

3.18 Neglected shoe rub. This large blister was caused by a shoe rubbing on an ischaemic foot of a diabetic patient.

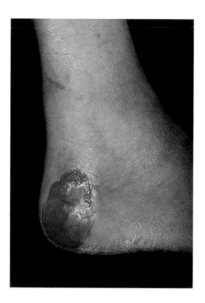

3.19A An ischaemic ulcer on the apex of the 1st toe. The lesion is partly covered with yellowish, closely adherent slough.
3.19B The same patient: the ulcer has healed following angioplasty.

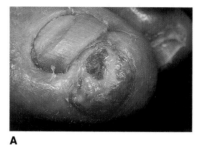
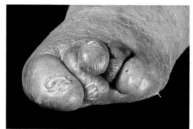

A　　　　　　　　　　　**B**

3.20 Ischaemic ulcer. A small ischaemic ulcer on the medial border of the foot in a patient with hallux valgus. This lesion looks small and innocuous, but it is a portal of entry for infection and should be taken seriously.

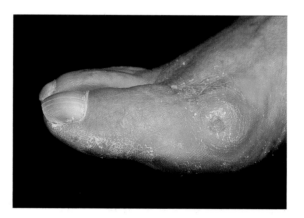

3.21 Rapid deterioration of ischaemic ulcer. This is the foot of a diabetic ischaemic patient who developed a small ulcer over a prominent hallux valgus and did not seek treatment. Infection set in and within 48 hours the small ulcer was 2 cm in diameter. The foot healed after an angioplasty and a course of intravenous antibiotics.

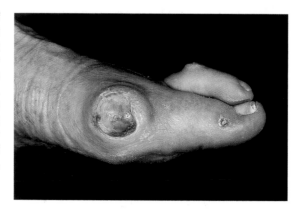

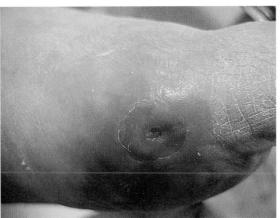
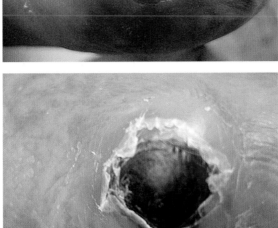

A

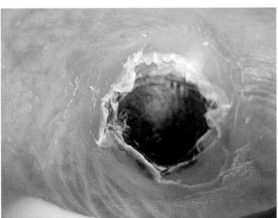

B

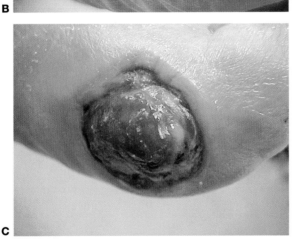

C

3.22A Early ischaemic ulcer. The foot is cold and pink and painful and this diabetic patient has been wearing a slip-on shoe, which put pressure on the vulnerable margins of the foot. This ulcer began as a tiny 1 mm blister that broke down. The base is ominously dark. The lesion looks superficial, but early ischaemic ulcers are very deceptive. Any breakdown on the skin of an ischaemic foot needs careful assessment and aggressive treatment.

3.22B This is the same ischaemic lesion on the border of the foot that presented 1 week earlier as a 1 mm lesion with a darkish base. Now the base is necrotic and the lesion has enlarged to 2 cm.

3.22C She underwent urgent angioplasty. Initially the effect was marginal, but after 4 weeks the wound was granulating well, as shown here.

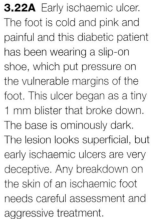

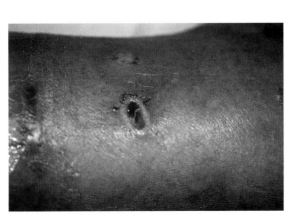

3.23 Ischaemic ulcer. This is a cold, pink, ischaemic limb with a small ischaemic ulcer.

3.24A Ischaemic ulcer. A small ischaemic ulcer on the medial border of the forefoot of a diabetic patient. The lesion is small and pale and surrounded by a halo of dry skin.

3.24B The ischaemic ulcer has been sharp debrided by a podiatrist. The halo of dry tissue has been debrided away to reveal the true dimensions of the lesion and to prevent the dressings catching on the halo and causing trauma. No injury has been caused to vulnerable ischaemic tissues by the debridement, which was performed very carefully with a scalpel.

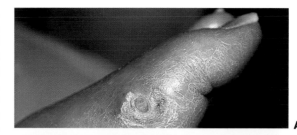

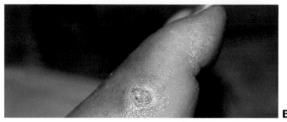

3.25 Subungual ischaemic ulcer. This 80-year-old lady with severe peripheral vascular disease – she smoked 30 cigarettes per day – presented with neglected toe nails and pain in the right 1st toe. The nail was cut back and a small ulcer was revealed. Her ankle brachial pressure index was 0.40. She underwent angioplasty and the toe healed in 5 weeks. Even a small ulcer, if neglected, can lead to loss of the leg, and apparently trivial foot ulcers should never be underestimated, as they need aggressive treatment.

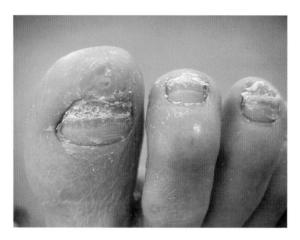

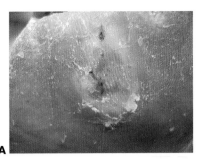

A

3.26A Painful ischaemic foot pre-debridement. This diabetic patient with peripheral vascular disease presented as an emergency, complaining of pain. Callus and plantar ulcers are quite uncommon in the ischaemic foot. On examination there was an area of moist plantar callus, but it was difficult to see the extent of the problem.

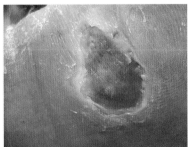

B

3.26B Painful ischaemic foot post-debridement. The same foot was very carefully debrided to avoid causing damage to ischaemic tissues. Removal of the plaque of thin glassy callus revealed superficial ulceration on the plantar surface. Examination of the patient's shoe revealed a rough place on the insole corresponding with the site of callus. The insole was replaced and the patient advised to check the shoes regularly. The foot healed within 1 month.

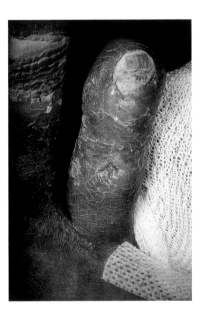

3.27 Healed ischaemic ulcer. This patient with peripheral vascular disease and cardiac failure had dusky feet, with numerous small ischaemic ulcers. This small ulcer on the dorsum of the second toe is now dry and healed.

3.28 Ischaemic ulcer in amputee. The remaining foot of a major amputee has developed an ischaemic ulcer on the border. The patient did not want vascular intervention and the foot is being treated conservatively with daily dressings and antibiotics. After 2 months, the ulcer is healing slowly and there is pearly new epithelium around the edge.

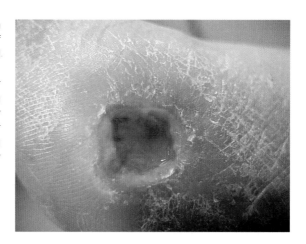

3.29A Ischaemic ulcer pre-debridement. The base of this ischaemic ulcer is pale and poorly perfused in this diabetic patient. The lesion has a halo of glassy callus forming around it. If this is allowed to continue there is danger that it will catch on dressings and cause trauma to the foot. Furthermore, if the glassy callus closes over the ulcer preventing drainage of exudates, the foot will deteriorate. Sharp debridement with a scalpel by the podiatrist should be performed.

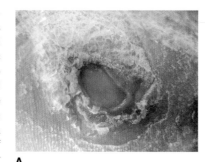
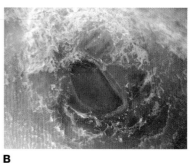

A   B

3.29B Ischaemic ulcer post-debridement. The callus has been debrided. The ulcer had been present for 4 months. The patient underwent angioplasty and the foot healed.

3.30 Rare plantar ischaemic ulcer with callus. Callus and plantar ulceration are commonly associated with neuropathy. This is a very rare presentation of callus and plantar ulceration in a diabetic patient with chronic ischaemia. She stood on a sharp object 2 weeks previously. Usually there is a history of specific trauma to the plantar surface to lead to such ulceration in the ischaemic foot.

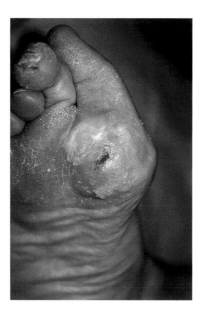

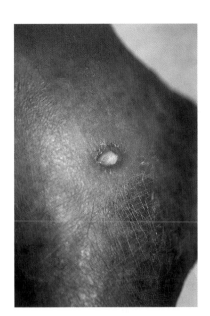

3.31 Small ischaemic ulcer on an icy cold, pink, ischaemic foot.

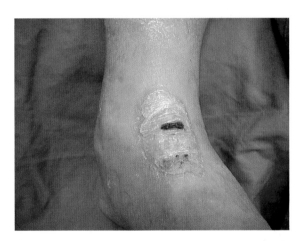

3.32 Scaling and callus formation around a healing ulcer on the front of the ankle of an ischaemic foot.

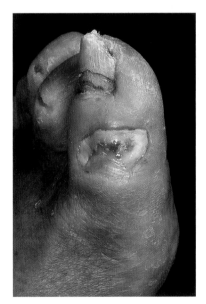

3.33 Improvement following angioplasty. Post-angioplasty, this diabetic ischaemic patient with an ulcer over the medial surface of the 1st toe is doing well. The ulcers are beginning to show healthy red granulation tissue, whereas before the angioplasty they were pale and very poorly perfused, with no granulations.

3.34A "Die back". After debridement, the adjoining ischaemic tissues around the wound have become necrotic. The 2nd toe is blue. When surgical debridement is needed in the ischaemic foot, then great efforts must also be made to improve the circulation by means of angioplasty or bypass. In this foot, the circulation is so poor that the patient cannot mount an inflammatory process (with its large vascular component) sufficient to heal the foot.

3.34B The patient has undergone angioplasty and the blue toe has been removed. The foot eventually healed in 7 months.

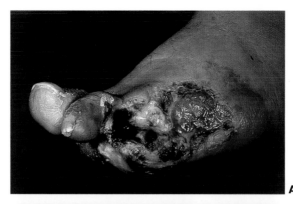

A

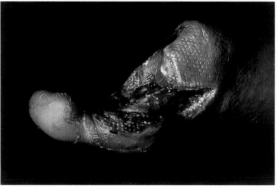

B

Necrosis

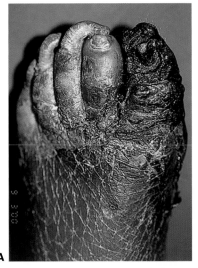

A

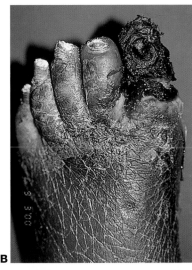

B

3.35A A sorely neglected ischaemic foot. The nails are long and have injured the adjoining toes. The foot is gangrenous. The patient was 87 years old, with dementia.
3.35B Same foot after debridement and nail cutting.
3.35C Plantar view before debridement.
3.35D Plantar view after debridement: note how much necrotic material has been removed.

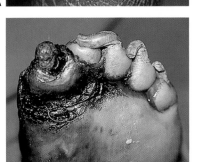

C

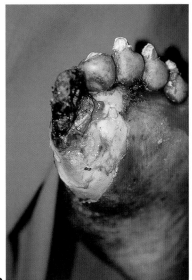

D

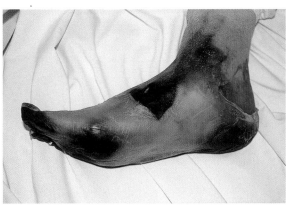

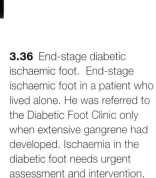

3.36 End-stage diabetic ischaemic foot. End-stage ischaemic foot in a patient who lived alone. He was referred to the Diabetic Foot Clinic only when extensive gangrene had developed. Ischaemia in the diabetic foot needs urgent assessment and intervention.

3.37A Ischaemia in the elderly. This 91-year-old lady has an infected 5th toe with bluish discolouration, necrosis and cellulitis spreading up the foot.

3.37B Close-up view of 5th toe. She underwent a distal bypass, the foot healed, and she lived for 4 years.

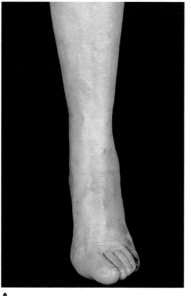 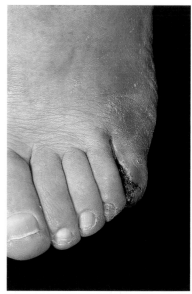

A   B

3.38 Untreated acute ischaemia. This elderly diabetic lady thrombosed her superficial femoral artery at home and her leg became acutely ischaemic. She had neuropathy and did not feel any pain. She did not seek or receive help for over 1 week. When she arrived at the hospital the entire foot and lower leg were gangrenous.

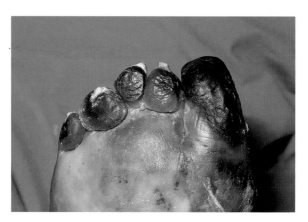

3.39 Necrotic toes. This patient has undergone distal bypass for an ischaemic foot. The next stage will be amputation of the necrotic toes.

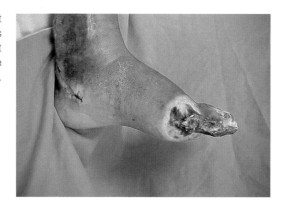

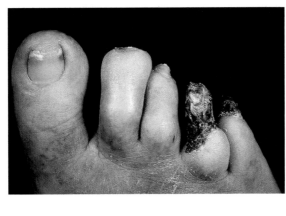

3.40 Debridement of demarcation line. This patient is receiving regular podiatry. The demarcation lines between gangrene and viable tissue are regularly debrided by the podiatrist, removing any debris or moist necrosis.

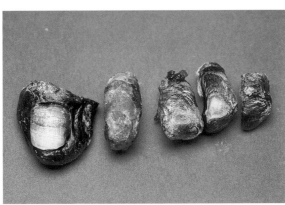

3.41 Autoamputated toes. Five necrotic toes from five different, diabetic, ischaemic patients' feet! All of these toes were allowed to autoamputate and all of the feet healed.

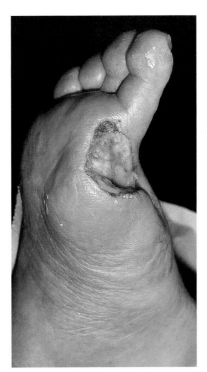

3.42 Dangers of corn cures. This patient with an ischaemic foot felt pain in his 1st toe and applied a proprietary corn remedy containing salicylic acid. The toe developed gangrene and was amputated. The resulting wound took over 1 year to heal. Revascularization was not feasible, but conservative care achieved healing.

3.43 Digital necrosis. The foot of a renal-transplant patient who was a heavy smoker of up to 40 cigarettes a day, but had palpable pedal pulses. She developed small areas of necrosis on several toes, which began as cracks in dry skin. This 1st toe became extremely painful and was amputated. The wound healed.

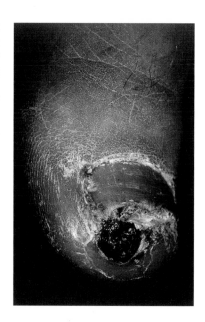

3.44 Dressing interdigital ulceration and necrosis in the ischaemic foot. This 72-year-old diabetic lady with peripheral vascular disease had an ankle brachial pressure index of 0.43 and no vascular intervention was possible. She was treated conservatively. Infection was controlled with systemic antibiotics. The toes were separated with dressings to avoid spread of necrosis from an affected toe to its neighbour. The foot healed in 5 months.

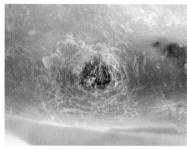

3.45A Necrosis predebridement. This diabetic ischaemic foot developed a small area of dry necrosis on the border, surrounded by a halo of glassy callus. It is impossible to assess the extent of the problem until sharp debridement has been performed. However, this should be conducted with great care to avoid inadvertently cutting the foot. Use of a scalpel and forceps enables debridement to be performed with great precision.

3.45B Necrosis postdebridement. Removal of callus and dry necrosis exposes a healing ischaemic ulcer. Note the pearly new epithelium and the small area of granulation.

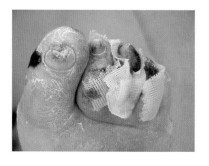
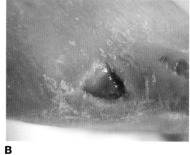

A

B

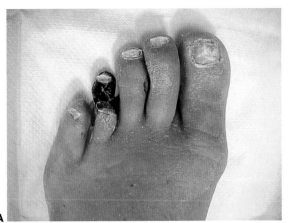

A

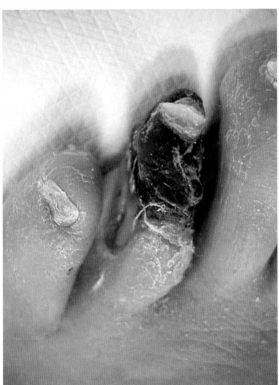

B

3.46A Demarcation line. Following angioplasty this patient's pressure index has risen to 0.63 from 0.72, the necrosis is dry and well demarcated, and the foot is no longer painful. However, the pressure index may still be too low to ensure healing if the toe is amputated. Antibiotics have been prescribed to render the necrosis dry and well demarcated. **3.46B** Close-up view of the toe. At fortnightly visits to the Foot Clinic, the foot was debrided along the demarcation line between gangrene and viable tissue, to debulk necrosis, remove debris, and reveal any infected areas. This toe successfully autoamputated in 4 months.

3.47 Extensive necrosis. This lady is 82 years old with diabetes of I2 years' duration. She suffered a stroke 6 years previously and is wheelchair bound. She lives with her daughter. Following an episode of severe infection, she developed extensive necrosis of the foot. Neither she nor her daughter wanted major amputation, although the lesion was extensive with exposed bone, and vascular intervention was not feasible. Pain was controlled with liberal analgesia, and she died at home of another stroke 2 months after being discharged from hospital, under the joint care of the Foot Clinic, the District Nursing Service and her daughter.

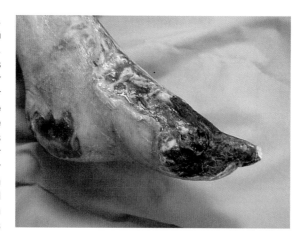

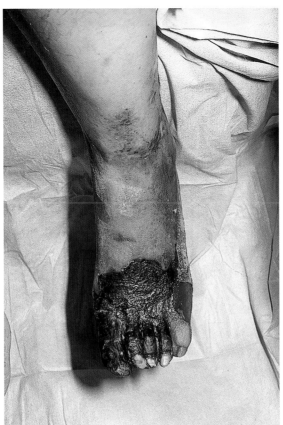

A

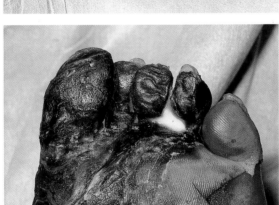

B

3.48A Extensive necrosis in diabetic foot. This was an elderly, Afro-Caribbean, diabetic patient with peripheral neuropathy and peripheral vascular disease, who lived alone and was occasionally visited by family members. He was not currently attending the Foot Clinic, although he was known to us from a previous episode of ulceration, but failed to attend for follow-up care after the ulcer healed. His family brought him to the Casualty Department after discovering that the foot was necrotic.

3.48B Extensive necrosis. Close-up view of same patient.

Emboli

3.49 Microemboli. These are microemboli. The macules do not blanch on pressure. Multiple deposits of platelet and cholesterol debris can embolize from atherosclerotic lesions and aneurysms in the proximal large arteries, so-called atheroembolism. This can occur spontaneously or after intravascular procedures.

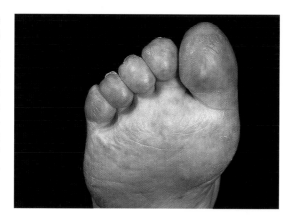

3.50A Emboli to the feet. The patient presented with painful necrotic tips of the toes.
3.50B Close up view of left foot.

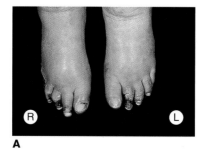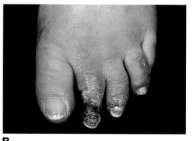

A　　　　　　　　　　　B

3.51 "Trash" foot. This patient has thrown off debris from an aneurysm in the abdominal aorta leading to trash foot, where thrombi have occluded vessels in the distal circulation, leading to gangrene.

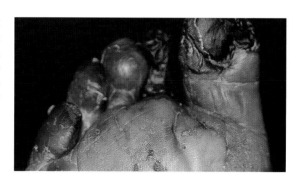

3.52 "Trash" foot. This patient developed "trash foot" with numerous small emboli, following an angioplasty for a stenosis of the superficial femoral artery. The lesions on the toes dried out and healed with no scarring or subsequent problems.

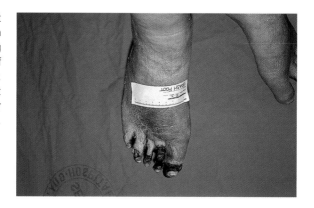

CHAPTER 3 Circulatory disorders

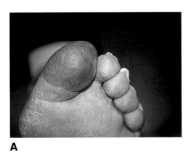
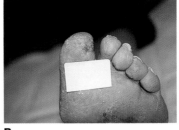
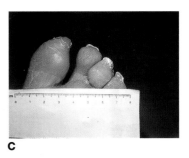

A **B** **C**

3.53A Embolus of the 1st toe. Often the extent of the necrosis is hard to determine at first. This first picture shows purple discolouration of the 1st toe; purple toe syndrome. As the necrosis developed, it appeared to be full thickness necrosis of the greater part of the toe. **3.53B** The foot has almost healed after conservative care and regular debridement of necrosis by the podiatrist. Only a small tissue defect remains. **3.53C** This final picture of the same foot shows complete healing; all necrotic material has been debrided away over a period of several months and much of the toe has been salvaged, although some soft tissue has been lost. The patient, a middle-aged man who lived alone, was a heavy smoker and found it impossible to give up despite referral to a smoking clinic.

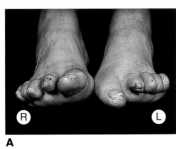
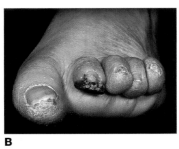
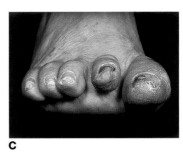

A **B** **C**

3.54A Embolus. This lady developed necrosis of the apices of the right and left 2nd toes after emboli, from an abdominal aortic plaque, lodged in her distal circulation. **3.54B** The left foot of the same patient. The 2nd toe has a necrotic apex. The necrosis is dry and well demarcated and was treated conservatively with regular sharp debridement by the podiatrist. **3.54C** Close-up of the right foot after a similar necrotic area on the apex of the 2nd toe has separated.

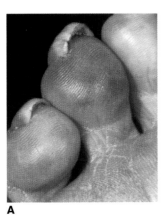
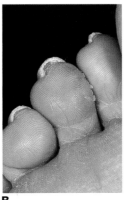

A **B**

3.55A Embolus. This lady threw off an embolus that lodged in an end artery of her 4th toe. Her peripheral pulses were palpable. The toe was so painful that she couldn't bear the toe nail to be cut. **3.55B** After treatment the toe is pink and no longer painful, and the nail has been cut.

3.56 Numerous small emboli.

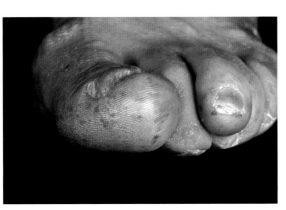

Venous disease

3.57 Varicose ulceration. This patient with varicose veins injured his leg when a supermarket trolley collided with him. He had developed extensive varicose ulceration 1 week later. Note the sloughy wound bed with islands of granulation tissue showing through the slough, and a small area of necrosis proximal to the main ulcer. He was treated with antibiotics and four layer compression bandaging and healed.

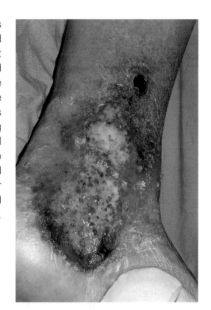

3.58A Varicose veins and pigmentation. The legs show dilated enlarged tortuous veins. There is pigmentation related to haemosiderin deposition. **3.58B** Close-up of the right leg.

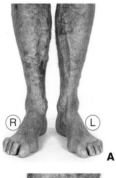

A

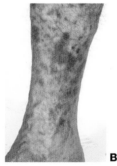

B

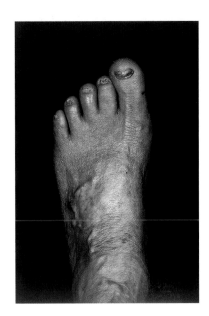

3.59 Varicose veins. This patient has numerous tortuous and prominent veins on the dorsum of the foot.

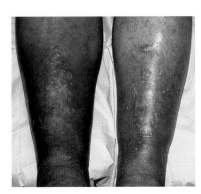

3.60 Post-phlebitic venous insufficiency. The lower legs show eczematous stasis dermatitis with painful brawny induration and broken skin.

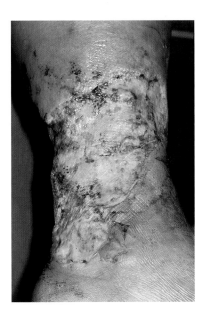

3.61 Venous ulceration. Ulceration in the classical "Gaiter" area caused by orthostatic venous hypertension.

3.62A Chronic venous insufficiency with haemosiderin pigmentation.
3.62B Healed venous ulceration with haemosiderin pigmentation.
3.62C Venous ulcer. It has sharply defined margins and an irregular shape in an area of pigmentation in the typical site for venous ulceration on the distal third of the leg.

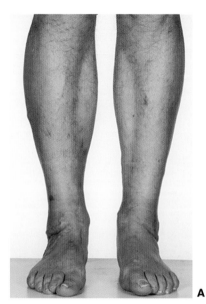

A

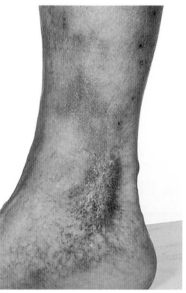

B

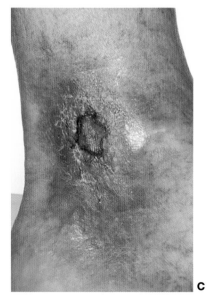

C

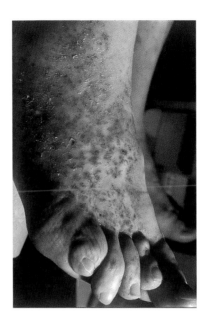

3.63 Atrophe blanche. There is atrophy of the skin resulting from poor vascularization and long-standing stasis dermatitis.

Lymphoedema

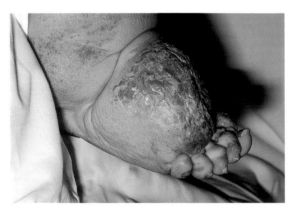

3.64 Lymphoedema. This patient has severe swelling of the foot, which is secondary to a build up of lymph. The patient had primary bilateral lymphoedema, which was congenital.

Perniosis

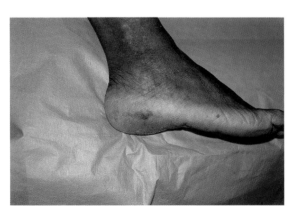

3.65 Chilblain (Perniosis). A chilblain has developed on the lateral border of the heel. The patient waited for a bus in cold, damp weather conditions. When he returned home he warmed his feet in front of a coal fire. The chilblain was red and intensely itchy. Injudicious warming of cold feet is a common cause of chilblains.

Revascularization of the ischaemic foot

3.66 Angiogram. This digital subtraction angiogram shows occlusion of the popliteal artery with very poor run-off into the calf. (Courtesy of Dr Paul Sidhu).

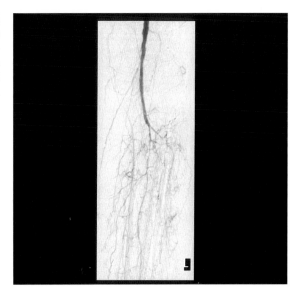

3.67A Magnetic resonance angiography (MRA). This shows the lower aorta and the iliac arteries, with a focal narrowing in the right external iliac artery.
3.67B MRA. There is diffuse atheromatous disease of both superficial femoral arteries, with an area of narrowing at the mid-level on the right. The popliteal arteries are severely diseased. (Courtesy of Dr Paul Sidhu).

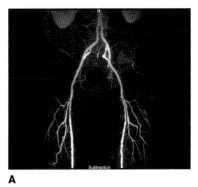

A

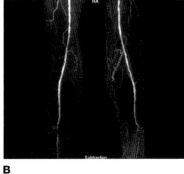

B

3.68 Leg wound scar and hypopigmentation. This diabetic patient with peripheral vascular disease underwent distal bypass. The leg wound took 4 months to heal. Also note the stocking distribution of hyperpigmentation. The patient is Afro-Caribbean.

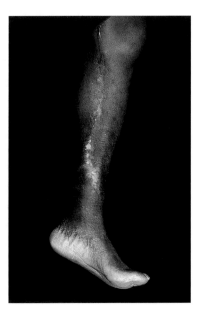

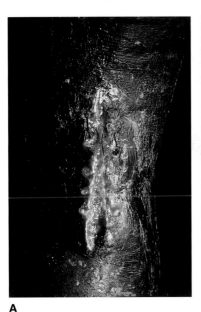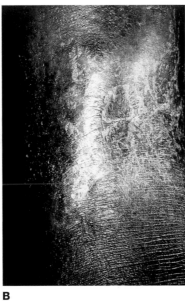

A **B**

3.69A Leg wound – healing failure. This is a distal bypass wound in a diabetic Afro-Caribbean patient. Eschar has been removed to reveal an area where the surgical wound is not yet fully healed. **3.69B** The same leg 1 month later. The bypass wound has healed. A strong pulse can be felt when the scar is palpated, as the new graft lies just beneath it.

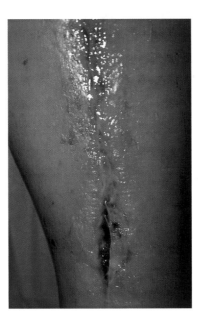

3.70 Breakdown of leg wound. This leg wound from a distal bypass has broken down due to infection in a diabetic patient. Careful follow-up of leg wounds until complete healing is achieved is of the utmost importance.

3.71 Early infection in a diabetic, ischaemic leg after revascularization. This leg wound from a distal bypass became slightly discoloured.

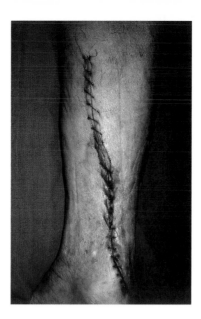

3.72 Broken-down leg wound following removal of saphenous vein for coronary-artery bypass graft. The leg eventually healed, but it took over 1 year to achieve full closure of the wounds in this diabetic patient.

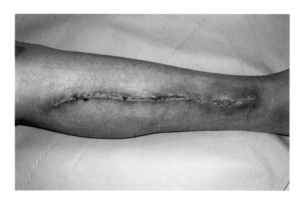

Nails

Introduction

Changes in the nails can be an important marker for systemic and local disorders. Optimal care of the nails is particularly important for high-risk patients, but nails in normal healthy feet will also become problematic if neglected, cut too short, or allowed to grow too long. The most common cause of an in-growing toe nail is inadequate cutting and care of the nails. Nails should be cut straight across, not too short and not too long. A splinter of nail should never be left behind, and patients should not poke or probe the sides of their nails. High-risk patients should be offered professional nail care. Malignancy and the nail are discussed in Chapter 8 (Malignancy). This chapter covers neglect of nails, nail picking, nail deformity, trauma, idiosyncratic reaction to cyclosporin, infection, ischaemia and differential diagnosis.

Nail neglect

4.1 Neglected nails. This elderly patient had poor eyesight and Alzheimer's disease. She was very aggressive and had refused domiciliary foot care for nearly 2 years before she was brought to the Foot Clinic and persuaded to allow us to cut her nails. No attempt should be made to cut nails like this in one piece as there is a danger of splitting the nail plate. Instead a gentle nibbling technique should be used.

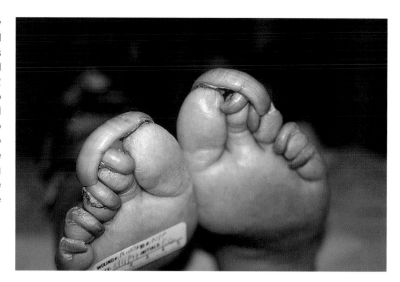

4.2 Neglected feet in schizophrenia. These are the 1st toes of the feet of a patient with schizophrenia who lived in sheltered accommodation. He was reluctant to accept care and was brought to the Foot Clinic at very irregular intervals. Even normal feet will develop severe problems if neglected. The feet have been washed and the nails have been cut and filed by a visiting podiatrist.

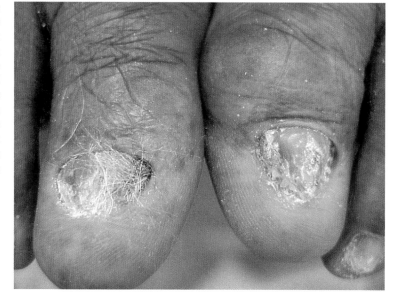

Nail picking

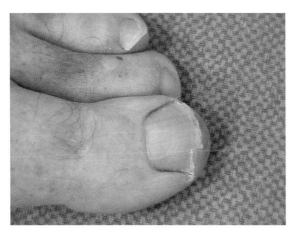

4.3 Nail picking. This nail plate is excessively thin and brittle. The patient is a young man in his 20s who, since his teens, has never cut his toe nails. When he feels they are becoming too long he picks at them and pulls pieces off. This habit can lead to ingrowing toe nails when a piece of nail is left behind and penetrates the nail sulcus.

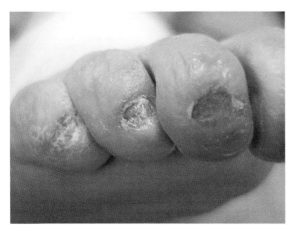

4.4 Nail picking. This patient never cuts her nails, but has a nervous habit of picking and pulling pieces off them. Because she has diabetic neuropathy there is no pain to restrain this activity and she has caused severe injury to the 3rd toe.

Nail deformity

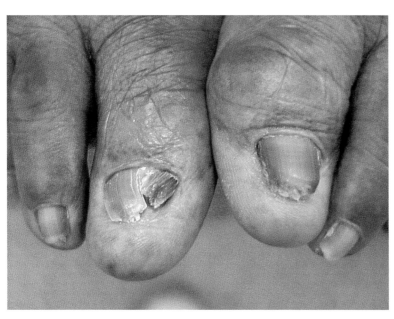

4.5 Onychauxis. Nails respond to chronic or acute trauma by developing thickening of the nail plate, also called onychauxis. This thickened nail has been cut too short and there is a danger that the free edge of the nail will damage the soft tissues as it grows forward.

4.6 Onychogryphosis. There is marked thickening and discolouration of the 1st toe nail plate, with less severe affection of the 2nd and 3rd. When thickening is associated with deformity, the condition is called onychogryphosis (from the Greek – gryphos = monster!) The old-fashioned term for this condition was "ostler's toe". An ostler was a groom and the deformity was common because horses would often tread on the groom's toes. Care is either palliative, with regular cutting, filing and thinning down by the podiatrist, or ablative, with removal of the nail and surgical or chemical ablation of the nail matrix to prevent regrowth.

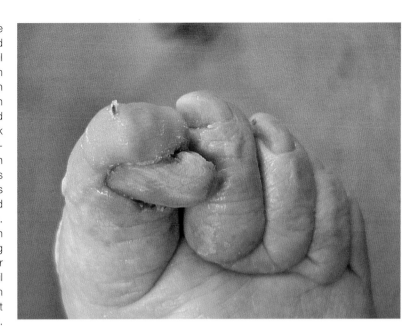

4.7A Onychogryphosis pre-cut. This patient has onychogryphosis affecting the 1st toe nail. Approaches to management include nail ablation or palliative reduction by the podiatrist.
4.7B Post-cut. The treatment approach opted for was palliative care and the podiatrist has reduced the thickness of the nail plate. This treatment will be needed every 3 months. In between treatments, the patient can use a nail file to reduce the nail if necessary.

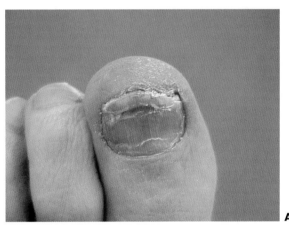

A

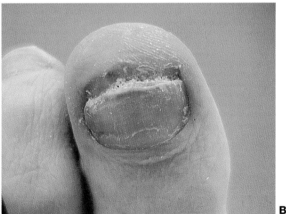

B

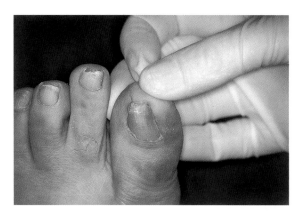

4.8 Involuted nails. There is excessive transverse curvature of this patient's nails. Unless they are regularly cut and cleared there is a great risk of problems developing in the sulcus.

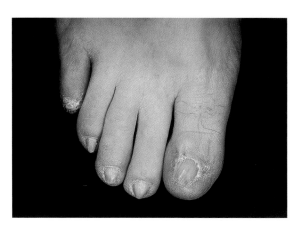

4.9 Involuted nail. The first toe nail is involuted, with excessive transverse curvature. These nails can be difficult to cut without causing trauma to the nail sulcus, and onychophosis – retention of debris, corn and callus in the nail fold – is a common problem.

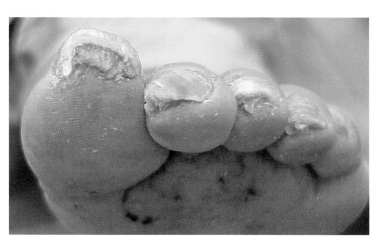

4.10 Nail tufts. This patient has nail tufts, which are bundles of keratinized epithelium just beneath the nail plate that contain nerves and blood vessels. The overlying nail is usually thickened. Tufts require great care to be taken when cutting the nails, as inadvertently cutting a tuft along with the nail plate leads to pain and bleeding.

4.11 Infected onychocryptosis. This 23-year-old patient had an in-growing toe nail, but did not seek treatment until redness, warmth and swelling developed. He purchased a proprietary remedy from the chemist but did not seek further help because he said the pain was not severe when he wore trainers. On examination there was severe cellulitis. A splinter of nail had been left behind when he cut his nail, and as the plate grew forward the residual splinter had been forced into the sulcus and had penetrated the soft tissues, acting as a portal of entry for infection. We prescribed amoxicillin and flucloxacillin, and removed the splinter of nail from the sulcus, and the foot healed in a few days. When managing onychocryptosis it is essential to remove any splinter of nail that has penetrated, or is pressing on the soft tissues around the nail.

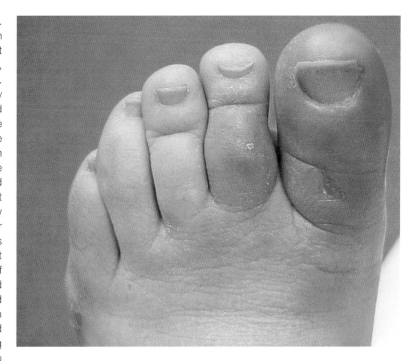

4.12 Partial nail avulsion follow-up. This patient was operated on 6 weeks previously for onychocryptosis. The nail had been a problem for several months, with pain and granulation tissue in the sulcus that did not respond to conservative care. A partial nail avulsion was performed under local anaesthetic and the troublesome area of the nail bed was chemically ablated with phenol to prevent regrowth. There was no subsequent relapse.

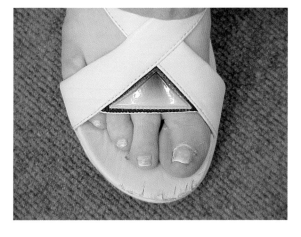

4.13 Onycholysis. This patient has a fungal infection (onychomycosis) of the right 1st toe nail that has led to thickening and discolouration. The majority of infections are caused by mould called dermatophytes or by yeasts, notably Candida albicans.

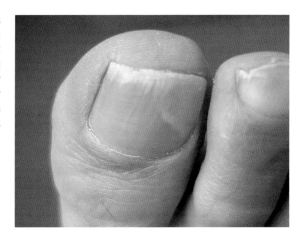

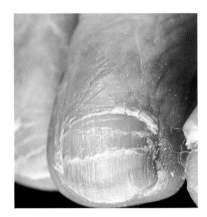

4.14 Beau's lines. This 79-year-old lady had a myocardial infarct 9 months previous to this photograph. This has led to "Beau's lines", where growth of the nail plate is interrupted by a severe illness or trauma.

Nail trauma

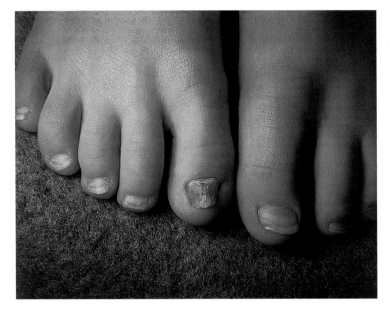

4.15 Onychomycosis. This patient has separation from the nail bed of the 1st toe nail plate. He had stubbed his toe 2 months previously whilst walking barefoot, leading to partial avulsion of the nail plate. However, the injury was not severe and there was no permanent damage to the nail plate.

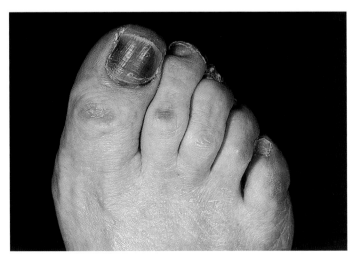

4.16 Sub-ungual haematoma. The patient walked barefoot and stubbed his toe causing bleeding under the nail.

4.17 Injured nail sulcus. This diabetic patient had painful involuted nails and used a tooth pick to try to clean out his sulci. He has caused trauma to the soft tissues with early infection of the 1st toe. The foot was ischaemic and the toe did not heal until he underwent angioplasty.

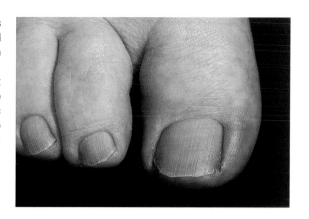

4.18 Very early trauma to a nail. This patient was walking barefoot by a swimming pool and caught the nail on a projecting piece of tile grout. The nail is loose and lifting, and there is bleeding under the nail at the proximal edge.

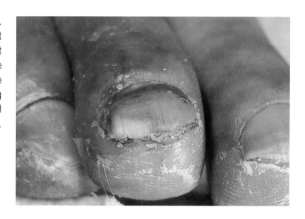

4.19 An old nail injury. The patient injured the 1st and 2nd toe nails by wearing tight shoes. He was 70 years old and felt no pain. His daughter noticed the colour change 6 months later, and thought her father had gangrene and brought him to the Foot Clinic. There are dry haematomata under the nail plates that are thickened.

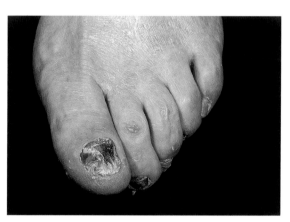

4.20 Trauma to nail. Following an injury, the nail of the 2nd toe is thickened and cracked. If it is not treated, there is a danger that the rough nail will catch on the patient's hose, causing injury, or that a thickened, gryphotic nail will press on the shoe, leading to a sub-ungual ulcer. The podiatrist cut and smoothed all the nails and reduced their thickness. This treatment should be repeated every 3 months.

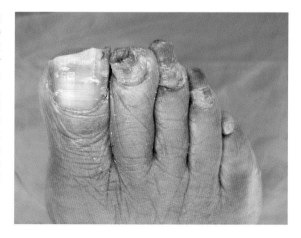

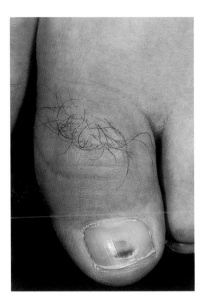

4.21 Sub-ungual haemaroma. When the haemorrhage is so small, there is no need to cut back the nail plate.

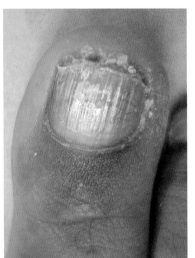

4.22 Nail plate trauma. The patient complained of pain and throbbing in his 1st toe of several weeks' duration. Careful questioning elicited the fact that he had bought new shoes around that time, with a narrower toe box than usual. The nail plate was subjected to pressure and rocking when he walked in the new shoes; the sign was the hyper pigmentation and inflammation of the soft tissues just proximal to the nail plate. A change of footwear solved the problem.

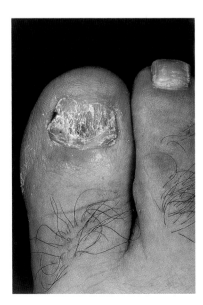

4.23 Traumatic avulsion. This patient was walking bare footed and damaged the nail of the 1st toe. The nail was ripped off. The new nail which grew was gryphotic (thickened and deformed) because of permanent injury to the nailbed.

4.24 Sub-ungual haematoma. This patient dropped a heavy object on his foot and developed sub-ungual haematoma of the 1st toe nail plate and fungal infection of the other nails.

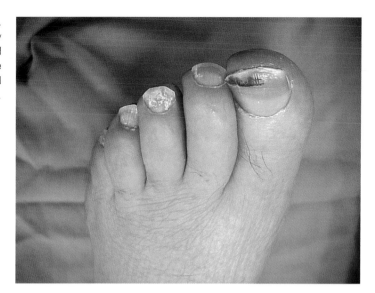

4.25A Loose nail. Following trauma to the 1st toe, the nail has become gryphotic and loose. If it catches on the patient's hose there is a risk of trauma.
4.25B The loose nail has been cut away without causing significant trauma to the toe. Regular reduction of the nail's thickness will keep the problem under control.

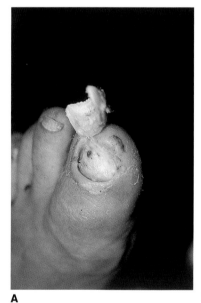

A

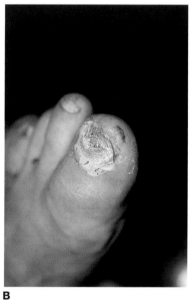

B

4.26 Draining a sub-ungual haematoma. The 2nd toe nail has been cut back to release a sub-ungual haematoma following a stubbing injury to the toe.

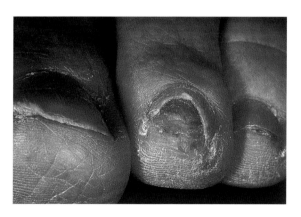

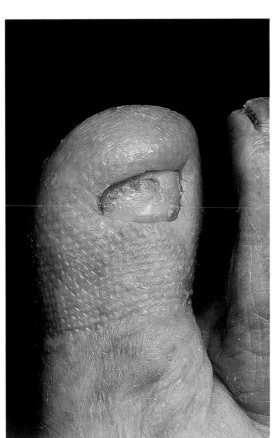

4.27 Successful total nail avulsion. Total nail avulsion with phenolysation of the nail bed results in formation of a fibrous plate.

Idiosyncratic reaction to cyclosporin

4.28A This is the right 1st toe of a patient with an idiosyncratic reaction to cyclosporin A. He developed granulomata in the sulci of all his finger and toe nails. Most of the lesions resolved with discontinuation of cyclosporin A, but the nail required removal and chemical ablation of the nail matrix to resolve the problem.

4.28B Close-up of the sulcus.

4.28C 6 weeks post-operatively, a fibrous plate has replaced the nail plate. The bridge of hypergranulation tissue has almost totally resorbed. **4.28D** The patient's left 1st toe; a lesion at an earlier stage of development. **4.28E** This patient was referred to the Foot Clinic as a case of in-growing toe nail. However, all his fingers were involved as well as the toes.

4.28F Close-up of finger nail showing granulomata.

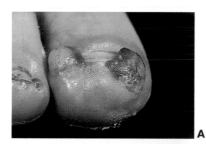

A

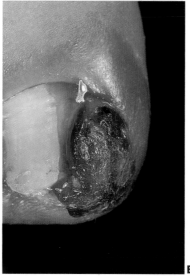

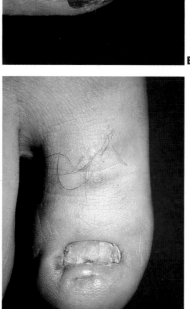

B

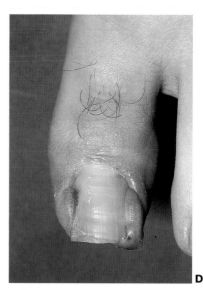

D

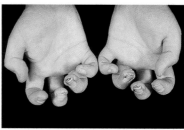

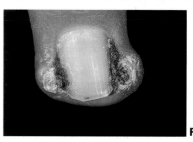

E

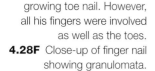

F

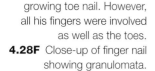

C

Infection

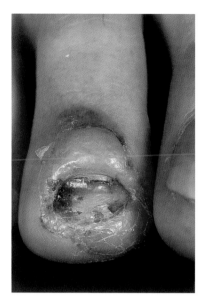

4.29 Periungual abscess. This diabetic patient dropped a heavy object on her toe 1 week before this photograph was taken. She has developed pain and throbbing in the toe and there is a fluctuant swelling just proximal to the nail bed. The nail plate has been removed. The swelling contained pus, which was drained as an outpatient procedure. The swab grew Staphylococcus aureus. The toe settled within 1 week on oral flucloxacillin.

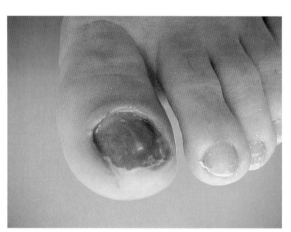

4.30 Spontaneous avulsion of fungal nail. This patient has a fungal infection of the nail, which drops off every few weeks. He refused treatment.

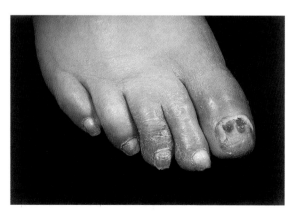

4.31 Draining pus from under a nail. The nail of the hallux has been cut back to drain pus. The toe was cellulitic and antibiotics were prescribed.

4.32 Fungus and trauma. There is fungal infection of the nails with areas of whitish discolouration, particularly marked on the 3rd toe nail. There is previous trauma to the 1st toe nail plate with thickening of the nail.

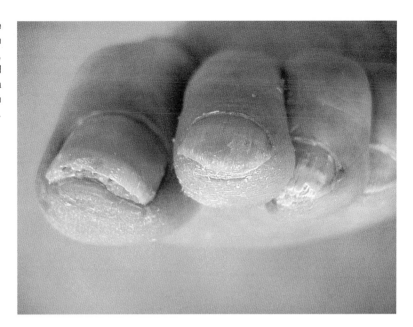

4.33 Onychomycosis. There is whitish discolouration of the nail plate. A sample was taken and sent to the laboratory for microscopy and culture. Fungal hyphae were seen and Trichophyton rubrum was grown on culture. The patient was very concerned by the cosmetic effect and was treated with terbinafine for 3 months. Onychomycosis of toe nails requires protracted treatment; palliative care, with regular reduction of the thickened nail plate and removal of friable material, coupled with topical applications of antifungals is a useful alternative to systemic treatments

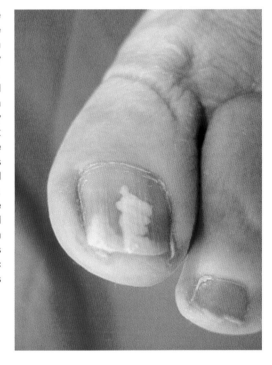

Ischaemia

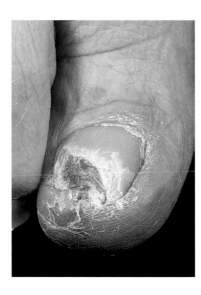

4.34 Sub-ungual ulcer. This diabetic ischaemic patient has a sub-ungual ulcer. The toe has such a poor blood supply that it cannot mount an inflammatory response to heal the ulcer, and the toe is turning blue. Severely ischaemic feet often do well until there is an injury. Even a small break in the skin can lead to disaster in these circumstances.

Differential diagnosis

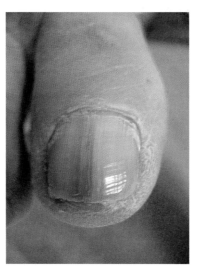

4.35 Pigmented nail band. This nail plate shows a small band of pigment. The differential diagnosis includes a malignant melanoma, and the patient was referred to the pigmented lesion clinic of the Dermatology Department and underwent biopsy. No malignancy was found. When the nail plate regrew there was an area of thickening, which was regularly reduced by the podiatrist.

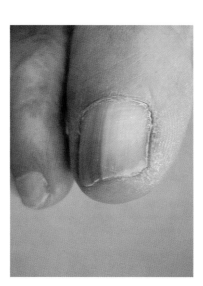

4.36 Pigmented nail band. Following an injury there is a discoloured groove in the nail plate, which will be a permanent problem.

4.37A Sub-ungual haematoma. This patient dropped a heavy object on the toe. There is bleeding beneath the nail and thickening of the nail plate. Sub-ungual haematoma may have a similar appearance to malignant melanoma and it is best to cut the nail back to ascertain the true nature of the lesion.

4.37B Sub-ungual haematoma, post-operative view. The nail has been cut back to reveal dried blood and an intact, dry nail bed. Subsequent growth of the nail plate is likely to be gryphotic and require regular reduction.

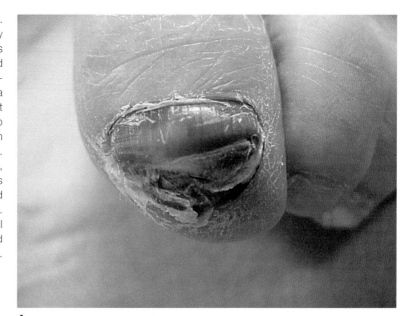

A

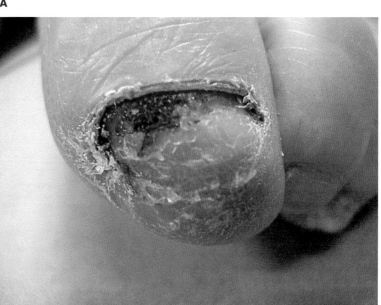

B

Deformities

Introduction

Deformities affect the structure and function of the feet and can lead to pain and ulceration, and even to the loss of a leg. Common foot deformities include hammer toe, mallet toe, claw toe, hallux valgus, hallux rigidus, plantar flexed forefoot, pes cavus, varus and valgus deformities and deformities associated with Charcot's osteoarthropathy, including rocker bottom foot, medial convexity and unstable ankle. Minor amputation frequently leads to deformity of adjoining toes.

Patients with deformed feet need careful assessment by a multidisciplinary team. The team should include an orthotist, as suitable orthotics, insoles, and footwear can successfully accommodate many foot and ankle deformities. This chapter includes mechanical, post-surgical, Charcot and other deformities.

5

Mechanical deformities

5.1 Deformity with corns and callus. This patient has claw 2nd toes with callus on the apices. The approach to treatment is two-fold; debridement of callus and relief of pressure and friction with suitable footwear and orthotics. Surgery can also correct claw toes very successfully, but should be undertaken with caution in patients with neuropathy or ischaemia.

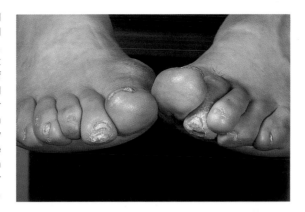

5.2 Hallux valgus, bursa and claw toe. This elderly lady has hallux valgus with a bursa, and claw deformity of the second toe with a pressure point over the dorsum of the toe. She needs special footwear to accommodate these deformities and prevent ulceration.

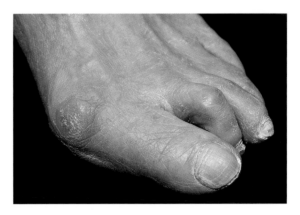

5.3 Trigger first toe. This deformity frequently leads to dorsal ulceration unless the shoe's toe box is sufficiently deep to avoid pressure on the toe.

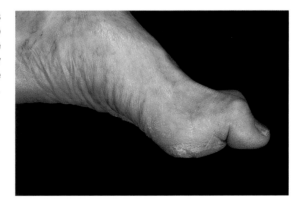

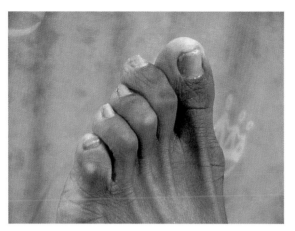

5.4 Claw toes. This patient has clawing of the four lesser toes. Note the prominent extensor tendons on the dorsum of the foot. This deformity may be flexible or fixed. Provision of a shoe with adequate fastening and broad deep toe box is essential to avoid injury to the dorsum and apices of the toes. If the deformity is not fixed then a silicone-rubber or felt toe prop manufactured by the podiatrist will improve toe function and prevent progression of the deformity.

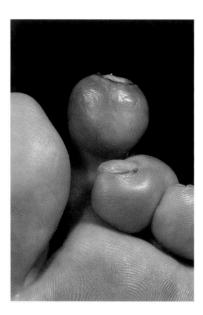

5.5 Overriding toe. The 2nd toe in this ischaemic foot is overriding and has developed a reddened pressure point over the apex.

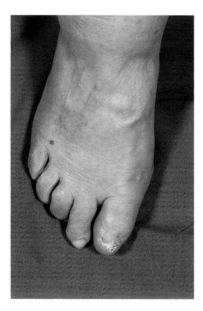

5.6 Digital deformity. There is medial rotation and displacement of the distal phalanx of the 2nd toe, and clawing of 3rd and 4th toes.

5.7 Flexible toe deformities in a young patient with ankylosing spondylitis.

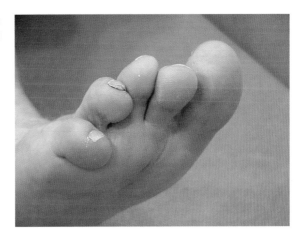

5.8 Deformity and callus. Following a previous episode of severe sepsis and surgical debridement, the patient's 5th toe is retracted. This has led to overloading of the plantar area with callus formation. The callus has been sharp debrided, revealing a pre-ulcerative injury to the underlying tissues.

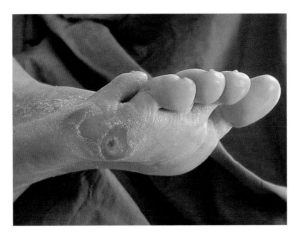

5.9 Cavoid foot. This common deformity leads to areas of high pressure on the sole of the foot as the raising of the medial longitudinal arch reduces the area of the sole in contact with the ground. A severely cavoid foot can be difficult to accommodate in high street footwear. This patient's ill-fitting boot has caused a rub on his ankle. A bespoke boot with cradled insole solved the problem.

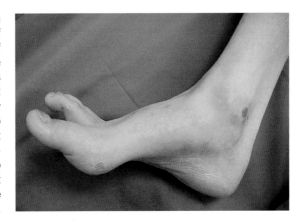

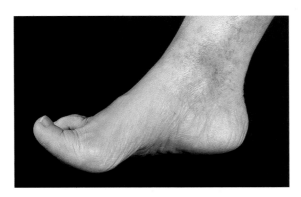

5.10 Deformity associated with neuropathy. Raised medial longitudinal arch and dorsiflexed 1st toe in a diabetic patient with peripheral neuropathy.

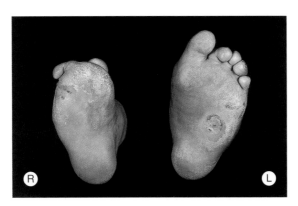

5.11 Diabetic neuropathy and foot deformity. This 44-year-old man has been diabetic since the age of 14 and developed his first neuropathic ulcer at the age of 26. He worked as a school janitor and had severe neuropathy. On the right foot the 3rd, 4th and 5th toes have been amputated, the 2nd toe has drifted laterally and the 1st toe is dorsally displaced. He has had intermittent neuropathic ulcerations over the 1st and 4th metatarsal heads for many years. The left foot developed Charcot's osteoarthropathy with loss of arch and rocker bottom deformity leading to callus formation.

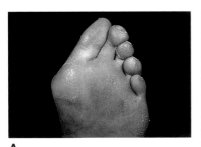

A

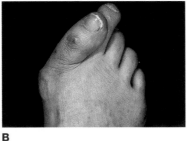

B

5.12A Hallux valgus.
5.12B Dorsal view of the same foot. The displaced 1st toe is over-riding the second toe. There is an adventitious bursa on the dorsum of the 1st toe where the shoe has rubbed the foot, and a small ulcer is present.

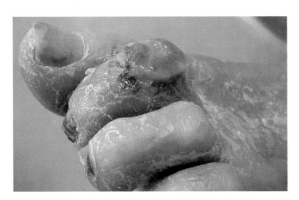

5.13 Deformity ulcer and infection. This patient had claw toe deformity and wore shoes with a shallow toe box, which pressed on the dorsum of the 2nd toe. A blister was caused, which ulcerated and became secondarily infected. If the deformity had been accommodated in a shoe with a suitable toe box, it is unlikely that this problem would have developed.

5.14 Bilateral hallux valgus. The right foot is cellulitic. The portal of entry for infection was an interdigital ulcer.

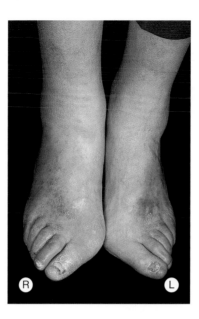

5.15 Hammer toe and tissue breakdown. Close-up view of a hammer toe in an elderly lady who wore slip-on shoes. She has a breakdown on the apex of the toe and a pressure point over the dorsum.

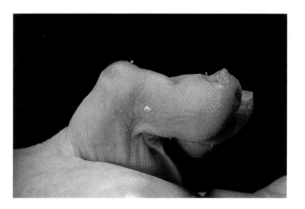

5.16 Deformity and ulcer in the ischaemic foot. There is clawing and medial displacement of the 2nd toe leading to shoe pressure and ulcer on the dorsum of the 2nd toe of this cold pink foot. Pedal pulses are impalpable. The ulcer is minute, but it is a portal of entry for infection and the patient needs urgent vascular assessment.

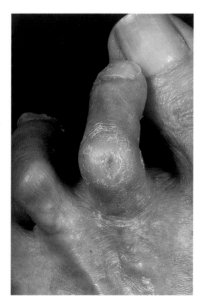

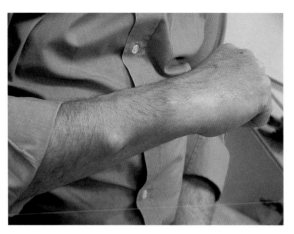

5.17 Ganglion. This patient has a large ganglion on the forearm. When these lesions develop on the dorsum of the foot they often require surgical removal, as it is difficult to accommodate them in normal footwear. Use of a family bible is not recommended.

Post-operative deformities

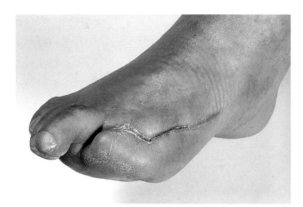

5.18 Faraboeuf operation. This is a procedure for removal of 1st toe and adjoining metatarsal head. If simple disarticulation of the 1st toe is performed then ulceration of the nub of the toe can be a problem.

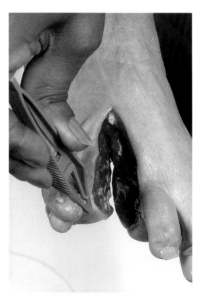

5.19 Ray amputation. This lady with neuropathic feet and bounding pulses developed gangrene after a neuropathic ulcer became infected. The toe and associated metatarsal head were removed in a procedure known as ray amputation, pioneered at King's College Hospital in the 1940s. She died suddenly of a myocardial infarction 2 weeks after this photograph was taken.

5.20 Ray amputation. This diabetic patient has undergone ray amputation for wet gangrene of the 3rd toe and osteomyelitis of the adjoining metatarsal head.

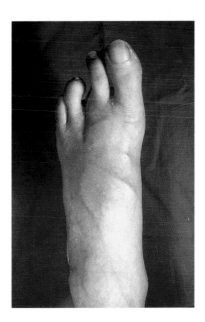

5.21 Ray amputation and incipient ulcer. This patient underwent amputation of the 2nd ray of the right foot. The scar is subjected to pressure when the patient walks and has developed heavy callus. Bespoke shoes fitted with cradled insoles, and regular podiatry to debride callus should prevent recurrence.

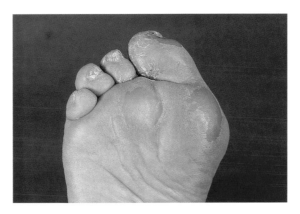

5.22 Ray amputation. This man was an undiagnosed diabetic patient with severe peripheral neuropathy, who presented late with two gangrenous toes. He underwent ray amputation of the 3rd and 4th toes, and parts of the adjoining 3rd and 4th metatarsals.

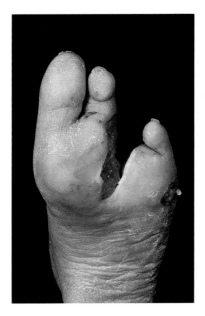

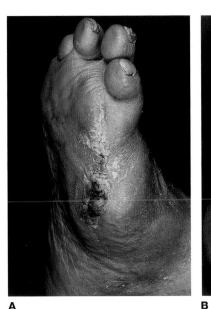
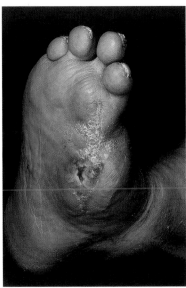

A

B

5.23A Post-surgery ulceration. This patient with neuropathy, who had undergone an extensive surgical debridement with amputation of the 1st toe, was lost to follow-up for several months and developed heavy callus over the surgical scar.
5.23B Removal of callus revealed a neuropathic ulcer. Post surgery, patients with neuropathy benefit from close follow-up in a Foot Clinic.

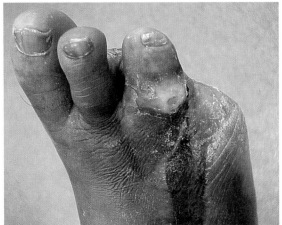

5.24 Post-surgery deformity and ulceration. This young man with diabetes mellitus and peripheral neuropathy first presented at the Foot Clinic very late, with extensive infection and wet gangrene. He underwent amputation of the 4th ray and 5th toe and skin grafting, after which he was lost to follow-up for several months. He returned to the Foot Clinic 6 months later. The 3rd toe had rotated and developed ulceration, and an X-ray revealed osteomyelitis. The toe was amputated and he was issued with surgical shoes with a filler and did not develop subsequent ulceration.

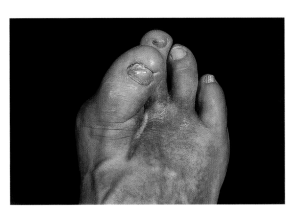

5.25 Post-surgical deformity. This patient with diabetic neuropathy underwent amputation of the 2nd toe for wet gangrene. The wound has healed 6 months later, but the 1st toe is drifting laterally and developing a hallux valgus deformity. This could probably have been prevented by provision of a silicone-rubber prosthesis.

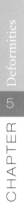

5.26 Amputation with sutures. This diabetic patient underwent amputation of the 1st toe for wet gangrene. The foot was neuropathic with bounding pulses. It was decided to close the wound by primary intention and inserted sutures. The edge of the wound was necrotic 1 week later and the wound bed was breaking down. The foot is shown after 5 months, following a further surgical procedure to remove all necrotic tissue from the wound, which is allowed to granulate from the base and then covered with a split-skin graft.

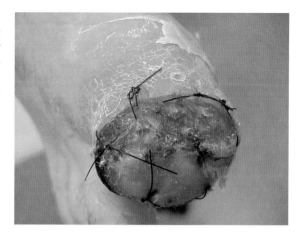

Charcot deformity

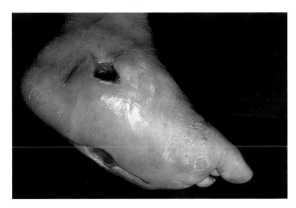

5.27 Charcot foot with rocker bottom deformity. Charcot foot after drainage and debridement for sepsis, and exostectomy to remove a plantar bony prominence. This is a rocker bottom foot in a diabetic neuropathic patient with end-stage renal failure treated by renal transplant. He was a middle-aged man who did not attend the Foot Clinic regularly. He developed neuropathic ulceration complicated by severe sepsis. He was admitted via Casualty and required surgical debridement, during which procedure the plantar bony prominence was also removed.

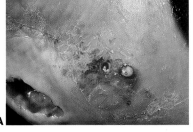

A

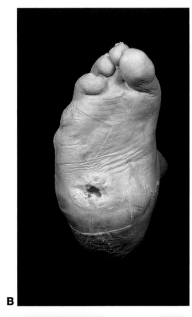

B

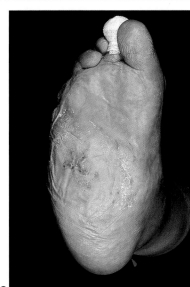

C

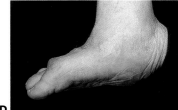

D

5.28A Spina bifida and club foot. This patient was operated on as a baby by Dr Dennis Browne and subsequently treated in Dennis Browne splints. He was first referred to the Foot Clinic, aged 58, with ulceration of 7 years' duration over a plantar rocker bottom bony prominence, having refused major amputation. Multiple draining sinuses were present, which discharged bubbly fluid when de-roofed, as seen here. He was treated with amoxicillin and flucloxacillin and fitted with a total-contact cast. **5.28B** The ulcer has improved 1 week later and all the sinuses have closed. **5.28C** He healed after 1 year in a total contact cast and subsequently did very well. **5.28D** This view shows the extent of his deformity.

5.29A Charcot's osteoarthropathy. This side view shows a medial prominence with underlying bone on the foot of a diabetic patient with Charcot's osteoarthropathy. The lesion has overlying callus, which contains blood and is an important sign of unacceptably high pressures that will lead to ulceration in an insensitive foot. **5.29B** Plantar view of the same lesion. The speckles of dried blood and blood blister are a clinical emergency. **5.29C** The same lesion after removal of callus by sharp debridement with a scalpel by the podiatrist. A small neuropathic ulcer is revealed.

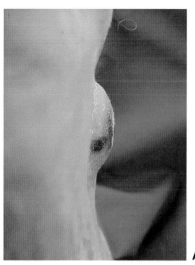

A

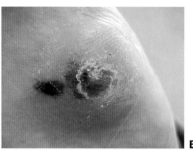

B

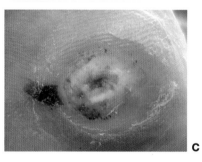

C

5.30A Foot and ankle deformity. This will sometimes develop with alarming rapidity in patients with neuropathy and sepsis. This patient developed Charcot deformity at the ankle joint over a period of a few days. **5.30B** Medial views of ankle showing new skin creases developing, which happens when there are rapid gross changes in joint position.

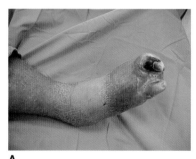

A

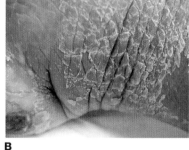

B

Other deformities

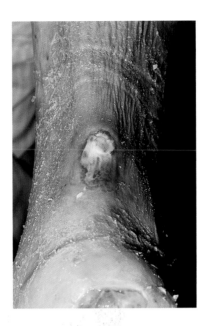

5.31 Ulcer over the Achilles tendon. The patient had recently had a stroke and became immobile. These ulcers are frequently slow to heal when tendon is exposed. This lesion was closed with Apligraf, a living human skin equivalent grown in the laboratory.

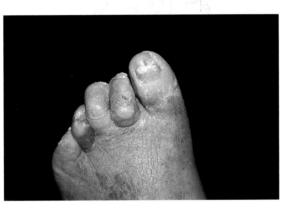

5.32 Deformed, ischaemic foot. This patient had numerous ulcers over the dorsa and apices of the toes, which all healed following angioplasty.

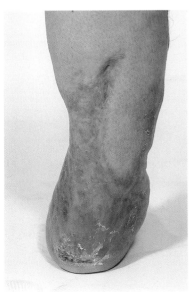
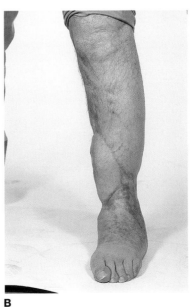

5.33A Free tissue transfer. The posterior view shows free tissue transfer to the leg of this patient who sustained massive skin and soft-tissue loss in a motorcycle accident. **5.33B** Anterior view of the same leg.

A **B**

Metabolic diseases

Introduction

Some of the worst problems presenting at Foot Clinics are seen in patients with metabolic problems. Liver disease, renal failure, cardiac failure, gout, as well as diabetes can all either cause or predispose patients to foot problems such as blisters, ulcers and necrosis. If oedema is present then foot lesions are likely and healing is impaired. This chapter will describe foot lesions in liver, renal and cardiac disease, as well as in gout and diabetes.

6

Liver disease

6.1A Wet necrosis. This patient had severe liver disease with ascites and had spontaneously developed numerous areas of wet necrosis on both feet and legs. Liver disease renders the patient severely immunocompromised and therefore susceptible to severe infection. **6.1B** There is necrosis of the dorsum of the foot. **6.1C** The leg is also necrotic. **6.1D** Spider naevus. Spider naevus is a vasodilation related to liver dysfunction. It is usually found on the trunk but this was seen on the dorsum of the foot in another patient with cirrhosis.

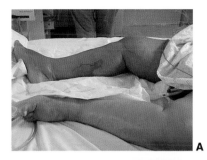

A

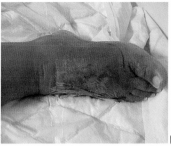

B

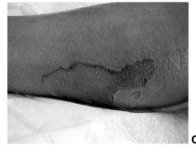

C

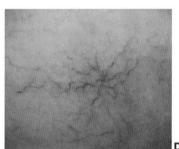

D

6.2A Group A Streptococcal infection in patient with liver transplant. This patient had a cellulitis with ulceration on the background of chronic stasis dermatitis. **6.2B** Healing of ulceration.

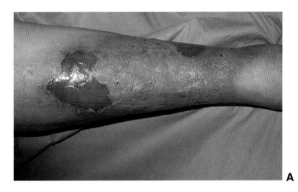

A

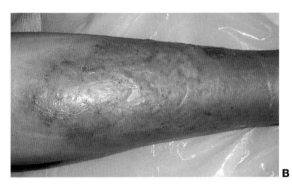

B

Renal failure

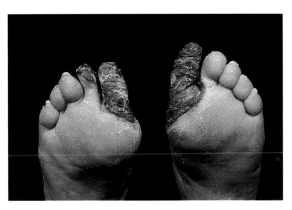

6.3 Dry gangrene. This woman underwent renal transplantation for diabetic nephropathy. She developed dry gangrene of three toes after wearing new shoes that were too tight. At the time she was a bowls champion and continued to play, winning a county ladies' championship and silver trophy despite her foot problems.

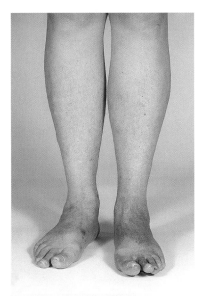

6.4 Bilateral oedema. This patient developed bilateral oedema related to diabetic nephropathy, which characteristically causes oedema early in the natural history of this condition.

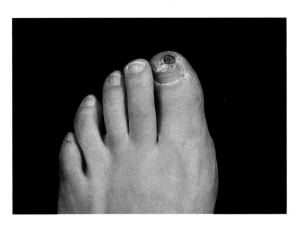

6.5 Digital necrosis in renal failure. The toe of a patient with diabetic nephropathy and palpable foot pulses. She smoked up to 40 cigarettes per day. The distal area of the toe developed dry skin and fissuring and a tiny defect led to superficial necrosis. The toe did not heal and was very painful, and the necrosis spread proximally. The patient stopped smoking. The toe was amputated and the foot healed.

6.6A Digital necrosis. This diabetic patient with end-stage renal failure, treated by renal transplantation, developed numerous areas of dry necrosis on both feet. She was treated conservatively with antibiotics and regular podiatric debridement. Her 1st toe healed in 5 months. She had no pain because of diabetic peripheral neuropathy. **6.6B** The left, 5th toe of the same patient developed necrosis following blistering from a shoe rub.

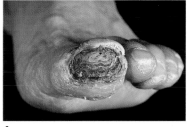

A

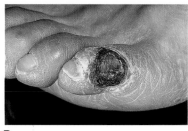

B

6.7A Early necrosis of a finger in a patient on haemodialysis. The digits – both fingers and toes – of patients in end-stage renal failure are particularly susceptible to developing necrosis after a small injury, even in the absence of infection and even when pulses are palpable. Vascular calcification is common in these patients, as are rheological abnormalities, both of which may predispose the patient to develop necrosis. **6.7B** Apical view of the same lesion.

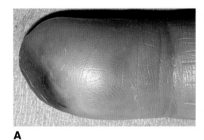

A

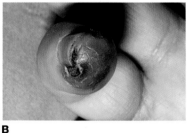

B

6.8 Necrosis of a finger in a patient on haemodialysis.

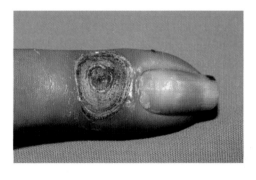

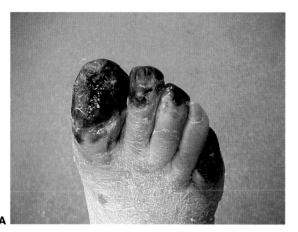

A

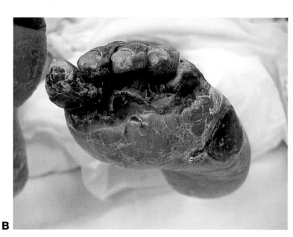

B

6.9A Digital necrosis in a patient in end-stage renal failure on peritoneal dialysis. This diabetic patient initially developed dry necrosis after attempting to cut his own toe nails. His pedal pulses were palpable. A small amount of discharge from the interdigital area between the 4th and 5th toes was detected, which was malodorous. A wound swab was taken and antibiotics were prescribed. On review 2 days later, the patient had decided not to take antibiotics and the necrotic toes were now moist and discharging foul-smelling fluid. The previous swab grew Staphylococcus aureus, beta-haemolytic Streptococcus group B and mixed anaerobes, sensitive to flucloxacillin, amoxycillin and metronidazole respectively. He was admitted for intravenous antibiotics and within a few days the necrosis was dry and well-demarcated. **6.9B** This is the other foot of the patient. It has also developed dry necrosis. The patient wished to continue with conservative care and not to consider major amputation, and he died at home, suddenly, 2 months after this photograph was taken.

6.10A Necrosis following trauma in renal failure. Necrosis in the feet of a 42-year-old man with diabetes and end-stage renal failure treated with haemodialysis. The problem started when he walked barefoot on coconut matting. **6.10B** View of medial border of right foot, same patient.

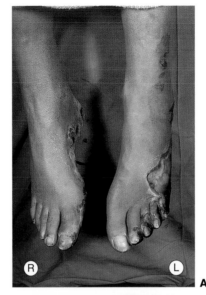

A

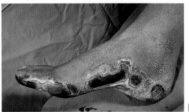

B

6.11 Skin problems in renal failure. This is the leg of a patient who had had a renal transplant 10 years previously. Skin problems abound in such patients; scarring on this leg is the result of removal of squamous cell carcinomas and basal cell carcinomas. The patient takes steroids, which render the skin fragile and prone to bruising. The patient is checked by the Dermatology Department every 2 months.

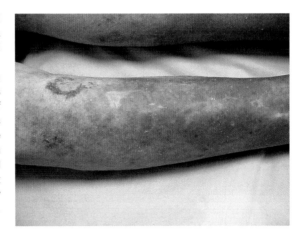

6.12 Skin necrosis. This patient, in end-stage renal failure due to polycystic renal disease, treated by haemodialysis, has a great propensity to develop necrosis after even a slight injury. The distal area of necrosis was caused when the patient pulled a piece of loose skin off the foot. Another piece of loose skin contains a small site of further necrosis, which has "shucked off".

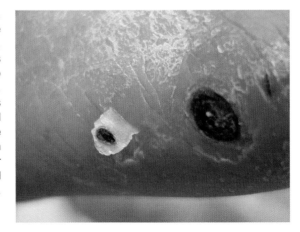

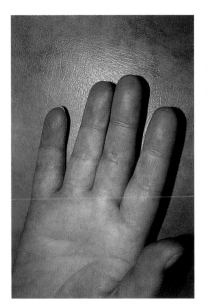

6.13 Ischaemia of the hand. This patient was on haemodialysis and developed acute ischaemia of the hand, needing angioplasty of the forearm arteries.

Cardiac failure

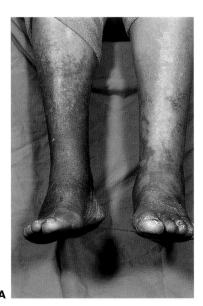

A

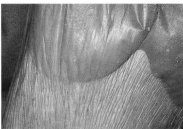

B

6.14A Ischaemia and oedema. The feet of a patient with peripheral vascular disease and cardiac failure are dusky and oedematous. It is essential to avoid injury to these very high-risk feet. **6.14B** Bulla. This large bulla developed on the dorsum of a patient's foot. This bulla was secondary to oedema related to severe congestive cardiac failure.

6.15A Oedema in cardiac failure. Severe pitting oedema of the feet and lower legs in a patient with cardiac failure. She was treated with diuretics and elevation of the limbs.
6.15B Close-up of the same patient demonstrating oedema of dorsum of foot.

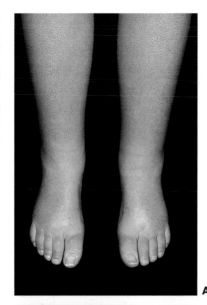

A

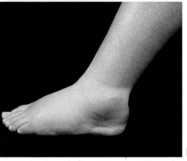

B

Gout

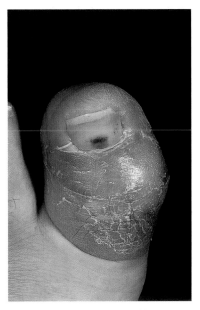

6.16 Gout. This lady crushed her 1st toe when she dropped a tin of baked beans in the kitchen. There is a small haematoma under the nail. The toe became red and swollen and antibiotics were prescribed. When the toe did not improve she was referred to the Foot Clinic. Acute joint inflammation in gout can be triggered by a trauma in susceptible patients.

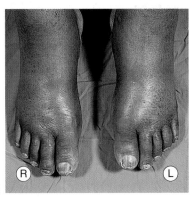

A

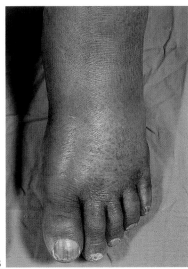

B

6.17A Painful feet due to gout. The patient complained of generalized pain in both feet over the previous year. He had previously had acute episodes of gout, which had now progressed to a chronic arthritis in the feet.
6.17B Close-up view of left foot showing oedema of the foot.

6.18 Gouty wrist. The tophi on this patient's wrist are due to gout. She takes allopurinol.

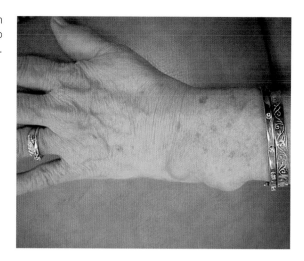

Diabetes

6.19 This diabetic patient has developed drug-related oedema following treatment with a glitazone.

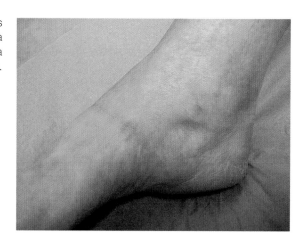

6.20 Diabetic oedema. Bilateral oedema in this diabetic patient was due to impaired renal and cardiac function, which often co-exist with diabetes.

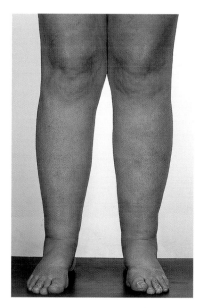

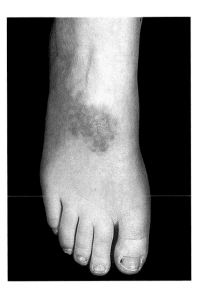

6.21 Necrobiosis lipoidica diabeticorum. This skin condition is most commonly seen on the shins of people with diabetes and its development may precede the diagnosis of diabetes by several years. It may occur as small waxy plaques or cover quite an extensive area, as on the dorsum of the foot in this patient. It is important to avoid trauma to the area as any injury may result in recalcitrant ulceration.

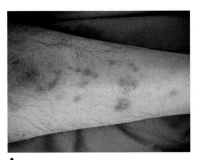

A

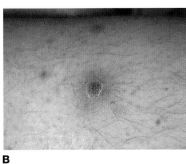

B

6.22A Diabetic dermopathy. These are chronic brownish circumscribed lesions, commonly seen on the front of the shins of people with diabetes. They probably develop after a minor injury. They are benign.

6.22B Diabetic dermopathy, acute lesion. This patient has injured his leg. The healing lesion is initially reddish, as seen here, but soon becomes a typically brown, chronic lesion.

Neuropathies

Introduction

In the United Kingdom, the most common cause of peripheral neuropathy affecting the feet is diabetes. Other rarer causes include congenital hereditary sensory neuropathy, leprosy (Hansen's disease), traumatic neuropathy, idiopathic neuropathy, poliomyelitis, spina bifida, amnion band syndrome and iatrogenic neuropathy caused by drugs.

Clinical presentations and complications of neuropathy covered in this chapter include inadvertent trauma such as burns, painless corns and callus leading to ulceration, neuropathic ulcers, rapid spread of infection, osteoporosis and pathological fracture, Charcot's osteoarthropathy and neuropathic oedema. We have included several pictures of the Charcot foot as we believe it is poorly understood and often missed, with major clinical consequences. Local treatment of painful neuropathy is also discussed.

7.1 Arteriovenous shunting in the neuropathic foot. Note the distended dorsal veins, a sign of arteriovenous shunting secondary to sympathetic neuropathy. The patient had a very warm foot, with bounding pedal pulses and dry skin.

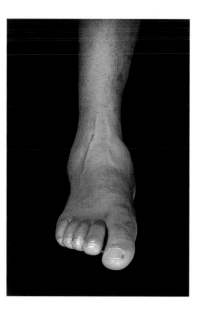

7.2 Distended dorsal veins. These prominent veins on the dorsum of the foot of a patient with diabetes are a sign of arteriovenous shunting, increased blood flow and peripheral neuropathy.

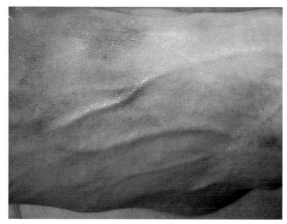

7.3 Neuropathic oedema. Neuropathic oedema is a rare complication of neuropathy and is diagnosed after excluding other causes of oedema. This lady with type 1 diabetes was treated with ephedrine, which was well tolerated long term and reduced the oedema. The dosage was 30 mg tds.

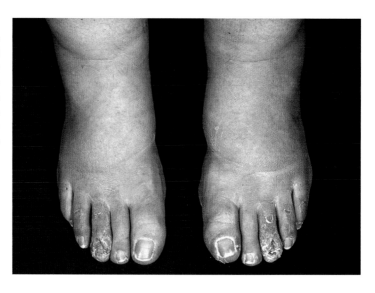

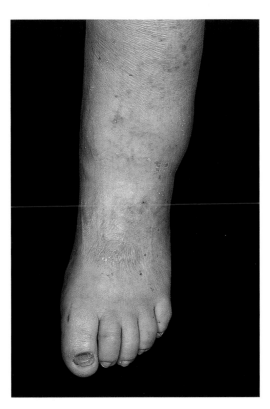

7.4 Neuropathic oedema. This is neuropathic oedema in a 55-year-old woman with autonomic neuropathy secondary to diabetes. It is often associated with other complications of autonomic neuropathy such as gastroparesis, diarrhoea and postural hypotension.

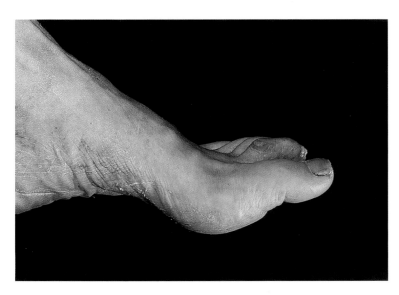

7.5 Neuropathic foot. This is a neuropathic foot in a diabetic patient with raised arch, claw toes and dry skin.

7.6A Callus pre-debridement. This patient with neuropathy has developed plantar callus. Note that the thickest areas of callus are discoloured. **7.6B** Callus post-debridement. Removal of callus reveals areas of whitish maceration and capillaries, which have been leaking blood in response to pressure from the thickened areas of callus. Both of these changes should be regarded as pre-ulcerative and an indication for emergency removal of callus. The only safe way to remove callus is by sharp debridement with a scalpel, in the hands of an experienced podiatrist, as chemicals that are strong enough to break the tough disulphide bridges in callus are likely to cause severe injury to normal skin.

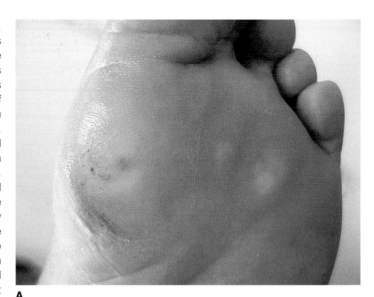

A

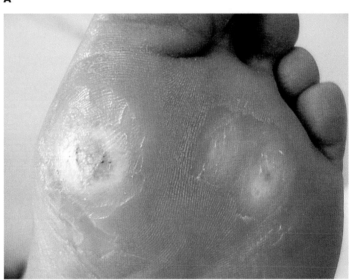

B

7.7 Prevention of problems in the neuropathic, post-surgical foot. This patient with neuropathy had an ulcerated 2nd toe, which became infected and developed wet gangrene requiring amputation of the digit. The wound healed, but 3 months later she was developing heavy callus over the 2nd metatarsal head. There was bleeding within the callus, which is a sign that ulceration will develop without treatment. A silicone-rubber prosthesis was made to fill the gap between 1st and 3rd toes, and to help to offload the 2nd metatarsal head. Over the next few months callus stopped developing and she had no further problems with the foot.

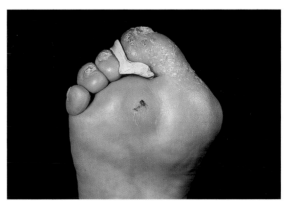

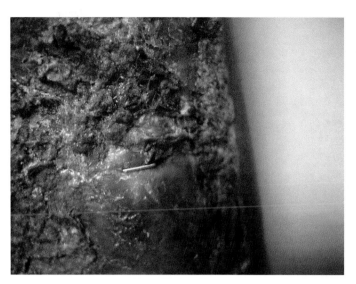

7.8 Foreign body. This neuropathic patient presented for a routine appointment with hyperkeratosis and a staple in his foot. He had been walking without shoes, which is not recommended behaviour for patients who lack the protective pain sensation.

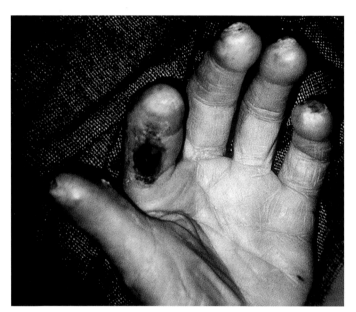

7.9 Neuropathy of the hands. This patient, with diabetes had profound neuropathy affecting his hands as well as his feet. He was a heavy smoker and lived alone. His hands were continually traumatized and he failed to apply dressings or seek treatment. Note the burn eschar on the palmar surface of the 2nd finger, burns and blister on the apices of fingers and thumb, and resorption of the distal phalanx of the 2nd finger. He was unconcerned – lack of pain led to "belle indifference". These are the most seriously damaged neuropathic hands the authors have seen in a patient with diabetes; however, many similar problems have been seen by us in the hands of leprosy patients in developing countries.

7.10A Burn on insensitive hand. Some patients with peripheral neuropathy of the feet also have insensitive fingers. This patient was a heavy smoker who had inadvertently rested a cigarette on the dorsum of his finger and sustained a burn. The burn was painless and he was unconcerned. **7.10B** The skin surrounding the burn is stained with nicotine.

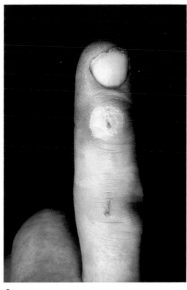
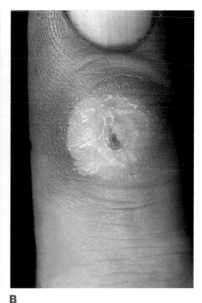

A   **B**

Neuropathic fractures and Charcot feet

7.11A Fracture and periosteal thickening. This patient had neuropathy and felt no pain from the fracture at the base of her 5th metatarsal. Warmth and swelling were detected and an X-ray revealed the fracture. The periosteal thickening along the shafts of the metatarsals of this patient is a common finding in patients with neuropathy.
7.11B The patient was referred to the Diabetic Foot Clinic 4 weeks later. The fracture had persisted and worsened. Delayed healing of fractures is common in patients with neuropathy, whose fractures take two or three times as long to heal as in patients with similar lesions who have no neuropathy. This patient was given a removable Aircast walker and the fracture healed in 5 months.

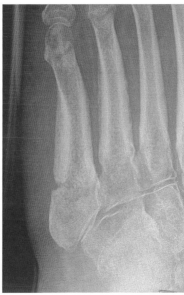
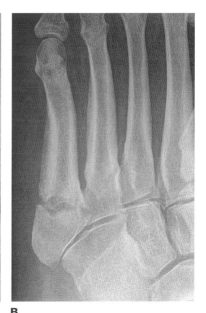

A   **B**

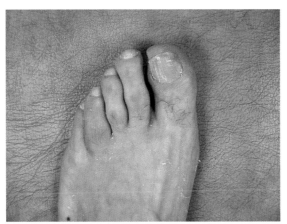

7.12 Fractured 4th toe. A patient with diabetic neuropathy presented with a swollen 4th toe. A neuropathic fracture was seen on X-ray. The patient was not aware of any injury; the swelling was detected at a routine appointment at the Foot Clinic. He had been walking barefoot and was advised to refrain from doing this in future.

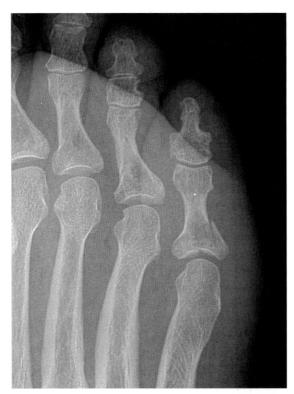

7.13 Neuropathic fracture. This patient with diabetic neuropathy was noted to have a warm swollen 5th toe. X-ray revealed a fracture of the base of the proximal phalanx. The patient was unaware of any trauma and said that he never walked without shoes. These lesions are very common when patients lack protective pain sensation. The patient was treated with a removable cast walker until the fracture healed after three months. Patients with profound neuropathy should have their feet inspected regularly.

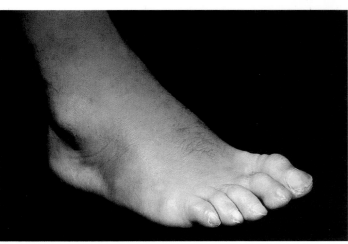

7.14 Acute Charcot's osteoarthropathy. This patient with profound neuropathy went on holiday and walked on uneven, cobbled pavements. His foot became red, warm and swollen 3 days later. There was no open wound or ulcer on the foot, so infection was unlikely. X-ray revealed an increased space between the bases of the 1st and 2nd metatarsals, which confirmed the diagnosis of Charcot's osteoarthropathy. He was treated in a total contact cast. When the signs had resolved he was given bespoke shoes with cradled insoles and did well.

7.15A A bruise heralds an early Charcot foot. The first signs of Charcot's osteoarthropathy can be subtle and hard to distinguish from soft-tissue injury following simple trauma. This patient with profound neuropathy had been taught to inspect her feet every day and come to the clinic at the first sign of anything unusual, even if there was no pain. She attended in emergency and reported a bruise on the side of her foot, as shown. The foot was neither swollen nor hotter than the contralateral foot and an X-ray was normal. As the clinicians at the Foot Clinic have a very high index of suspicion for Charcot's osteoarthropathy in neuropathic patients, the patient was advised to rest, a removable Aircast walker was applied and a diphosphonate bone scan was arranged. **7.15B** Developing Charcot foot. The bone scan, taken 48 hours later, confirmed Charcot's osteoarthropathy, by which time the entire foot and ankle was red, hot and swollen with distension of the dorsal veins. The X-ray remained normal.

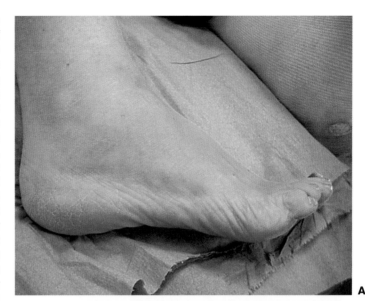

A

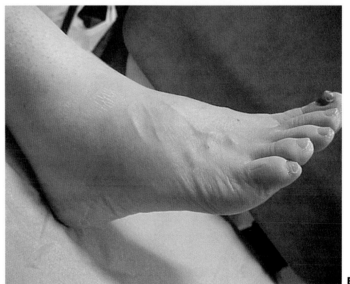

B

7.16 Charcot foot. Note the mid-foot changes with dislocation of the tarsal-metatarsal joints.

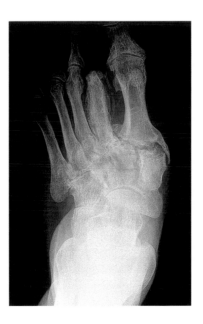

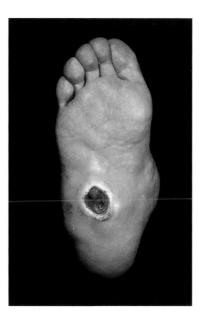

7.17 Rocker bottom, Charcot foot with ulcer. This patient was a professional chauffeur in his 50s who drove a non-automatic car and presented late with established rocker bottom deformity due to Charcot's osteoarthropathy. He refused to wear bespoke shoes because they were "not smart enough to go with the chauffeur's uniform" and developed a neuropathic ulcer over the bony prominence on his foot.

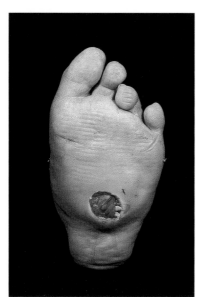

7.18 Charcot's osteoarthropathy triggered by surgery. This man with diabetic neuropathy underwent amputation of the left 3rd toe for wet gangrene. He developed acute Charcot's osteoarthropathy 2 months later and a deformed rocker bottom foot which was complicated by neuropathic ulceration. Charcot's osteoarthropathy is frequently triggered by surgery. For this reason, elective surgery should be approached very cautiously and avoided wherever possible if the patient has neuropathy.

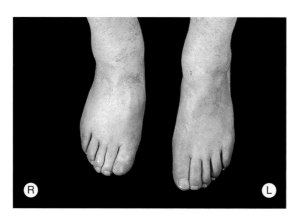

7.19 Charcot foot following restoration of circulation. These are the feet of a 64-year-old man with diabetes. He was previously neuro-ischaemic and underwent a distal bypass on the right side for critical ischaemia. The procedure was successful and he had strong pedal pulses. However, over the next year he developed Charcot's osteoarthropathy of the right foot. Its onset was very gradual and insidious, with minimal swelling and warmth, and the diagnosis was delayed for several months.

7.20 Incipient Charcot foot. This patient was treated for a neuropathic ulcer in a total contact cast. He remained in the cast for 2 months. After the cast was removed an X-ray was taken, which was normal. He was advised to rest, but instead he went to a football match. The next day his foot was red, warm and swollen. Patients who have been immobilized in a cast develop osteoporosis and too rapid rehabilitation can trigger a Charcot's osteoarthropathy.

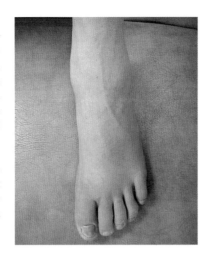

Non-diabetic neuropathies

7.21 Charcot deformity. This lady presented late with established deformity due to Charcot's osteoarthropathy. She is managed conservatively with hospital footwear and regular debridement of callus.

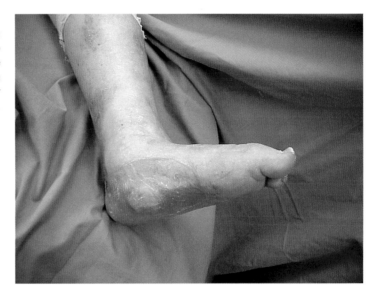

7.22 Hereditary sensory neuropathy. This lady had a hereditary sensory neuropathy. When she first came to the Foot Clinic she had already undergone amputation of the left leg for infected neuropathic ulceration, and had a deep plantar ulcer over the right 2nd metatarsal head and osteomyelitis of the 2nd toe. She underwent a ray amputation and the foot healed, but subsequently developed callus. However, she did well, attending the Foot Clinic regularly for callus removal and wearing a silicone-rubber toe prosthesis and bespoke shoes with cradled insole.

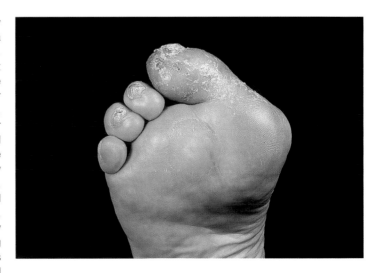

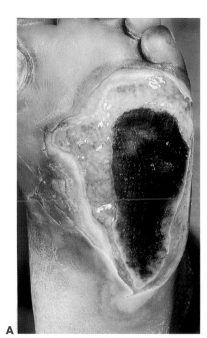

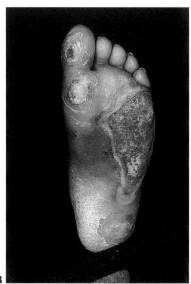

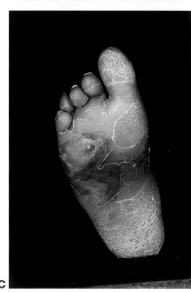

7.23A Idiopathic neuropathy. This patient with neuropathy suffered a severe burn when walking on the beach. The black area is a necrotic eschar. This photograph was taken on the day that he realized that he had a foot problem because of the odour from the infected burn.
7.23B Idiopathic neuropathy: the same foot after debridement.
7.23C The same patient, other foot showing healed ulceration.

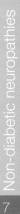

A

B

C

7.24 Leprosy. This patient has Hansen's disease (leprosy) with profound sensory neuropathy and a long history of ulceration and infection with multiple toe deformities.

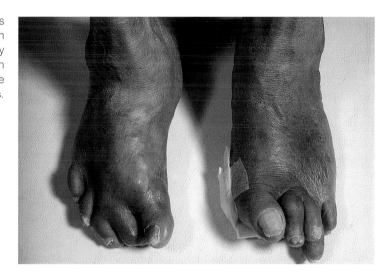

7.25 Neuropathic ulcer of the knee due to AIDS. This patient had AIDS (acquired immune deficiency syndrome), which caused severe neuropathy. He developed a neuropathic ulcer on his foot, which became infected, and he did not seek treatment until the infection was so severe that a below-knee amputation was needed. He was subsequently lost to follow-up until he presented with neuropathic ulceration of both knees. He had been unable to wear a prosthesis and had progressed around the house on his hands and knees. Because his knees were neuropathic, he was not aware that he was overloading them.

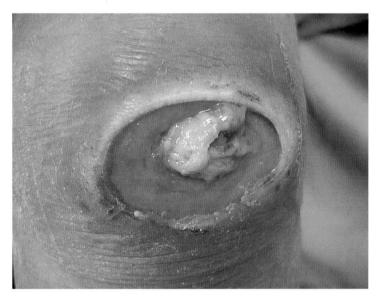

7.26 A neuropathic ulcer on the plantar forefoot of a 28-year-old lady with spina bifida occulta and peripheral neuropathy. She had two young children and found it impossible to rest and offload the foot. The base of the ulcer appeared to be clean, but close inspection revealed a sinus that probed to bone. Callus surrounded the ulcer, which is on a plantar pressure point overlying the 1st metatarsal head.

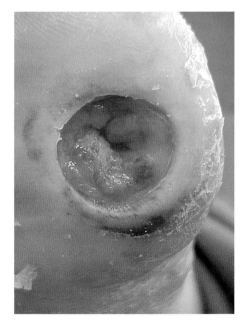

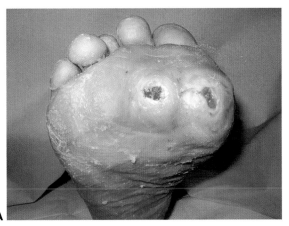

7.27A This lady had polio as a teenager in the 1950s affecting the right lower limb. She developed a plantaris deformity and walked on the forefoot with the heel never touching the ground. With increasing age, she developed pressure ulceration over the metatarsal heads.
7.27B A side view of the foot shows the plantar pressure points and deformity plantaris.

A

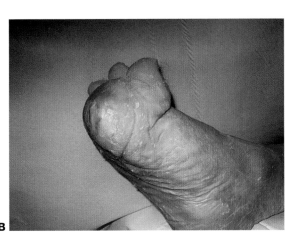

B

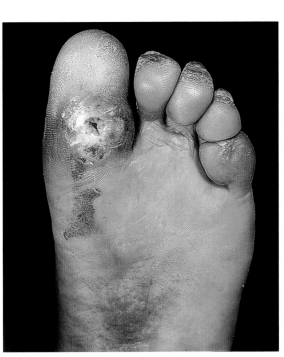

7.28 Traumatic neuropathy. This young man sustained three gun shot wounds to his left thigh. The sciatic nerve was severed and he developed profound unilateral neuropathy. Within 1 year he had heavy calluses and neuropathic ulcers. He developed 1st toe rigidus with overloading of the plantar surface of the 1st toe and a deep ulcer with a sinus to the joint cavity.

7.29A Neuropathy and schizophrenia. Neuropathic patients with concurrent psychotic disease can be difficult to manage. This patient had schizophrenia, was socially isolated, and failed to attend the Foot Clinic. He injured his 1st toe but did not seek help until gangrene had developed. **7.29B** Dorsal view of the same foot. **7.29C** His 1st toe was amputated. **7.29D** Dorsal view of the same foot. **7.29E** The same foot, almost healed. When he was discharged from hospital, the patient was offered accommodation in a sheltered housing development, where friends would check his feet every day and bring him to the Foot Clinic for regular appointments, and he did well subsequently.

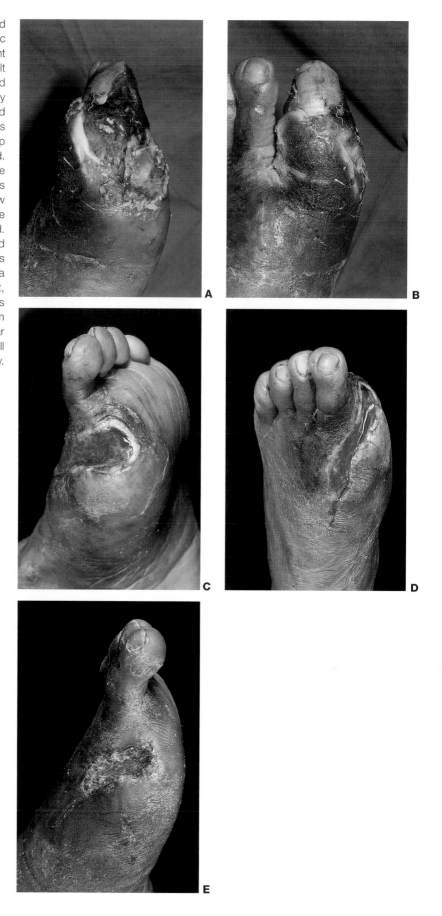

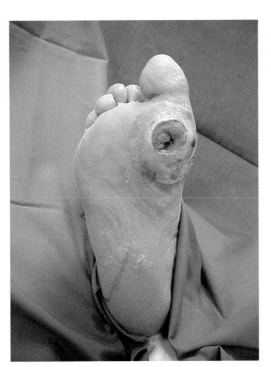

7.30 Drug-related neuropathy with plantar ulcer. The neuropathy was drug-related: the patient was taking Mesalazine for colitis.

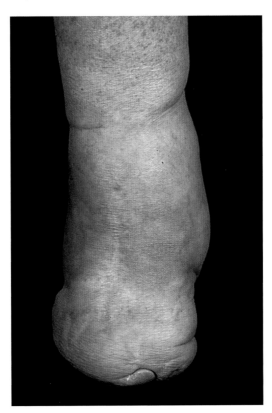

7.31 Amnion band syndrome. This patient was born with a constricting band around the right ankle, which appears as a deep groove leading to a deformed right foot. The amnion is the thin membranous sac that contains the foetus and amniotic fluid. Rarely, the amnion ruptures and fibrous bands from the amnion can wrap around the extremities and partially constrict them.

7.32A Treatment for a sacral teratoma caused a unilateral neuropathy. At the age of 7 years, this African girl was brought to the United Kingdom for treatment of a tumour at the base of the spine, which proved to be a yolk-sac tumour. After treatment with surgery and radiotherapy, she had profound unilateral neuropathy. At the age of 10 she went roller skating and came home with a blistered foot. The lesion progressed into a neuropathic ulcer. **7.32B** A medial view of the same foot; the patient had foot drop and had lost the arch of the foot, which led to overloading of the lateral border. **7.32C** After the ulcer healed, the patient was issued with an ankle–foot orthosis to offload the overloaded lateral surface of the foot. The orthosis was accommodated in a hospital boot. **7.32D** The patient did not like the cosmetic appearance of the orthosis and wore trousers to hide it.

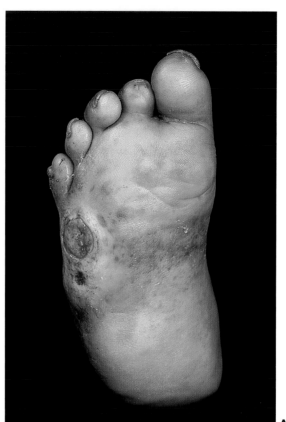

A

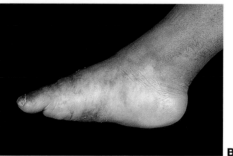

B

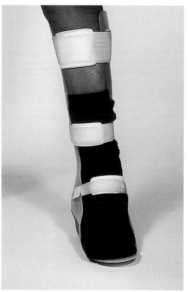

C

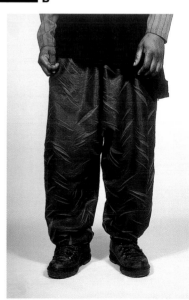

D

Complications of neuropathy

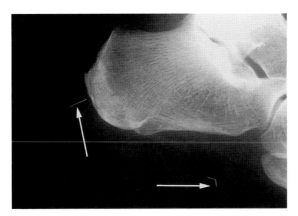

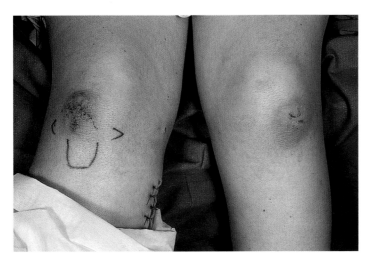

7.33 Foreign bodies. This lady with diabetes and profound neuropathy used a pair of wire cutters to clip off the sharp points from her insulin needles before disposing of them in the dustbin. She had a shag pile rug in her bedroom and some of the cut-off needles dropped into the rug. She was seen at the Foot Clinic complaining of pain and ulceration of the heel. An X-ray revealed two insulin needle ends deeply embedded in her foot.

7.34 Knee callosities post amputation. This neuropathic patient underwent below-knee amputation for an unstable Charcot ankle complicated by indolent ulceration and infection. She crawled on her hands and knees, and developed callosities on both knees.

OpSite treatment for neuropathy

7.35A OpSite treatment for painful neuropathy. This patient has diabetic painful neuropathy and complains of severe burning pain in both feet and legs, which is worse at night. He also has contact discomfort and "lightning pains", which are shooting pains like electric shocks. There are many treatments for painful neuropathy; this patient is having OpSite film applied to the painful areas, which is a simple, safe and non-invasive treatment.

7.35B OpSite for painful neuropathy. OpSite film has been applied to the entire stocking distribution. It can remain in place for 2 weeks and should be removed with great care.

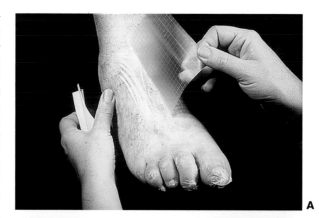

A

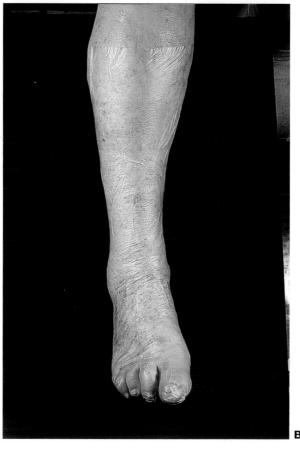

B

Malignancy

Introduction

Malignant tumours affecting the foot are rare, but can have devastating effects. The most common lesions seen in the Foot Clinic are squamous cell carcinomas, which may arise de novo or within an indolent ulcer or scar. Early detection is essential to save the limb and life of the patient with a malignant tumour, and Foot Clinics should work closely with Departments of Dermatology and Oncology. We have worked with both these departments when treating a case of mycosis fungoides, a singularly disagreeable invasion of the skin of the feet by lymphoma, leading to exquisitely painful hyperkeratosis, cracking and ulceration that needed daily debridement by the podiatrists to keep the patient comfortable. Malignant disease may metastasize to the feet; in addition, treatments of malignant disease may affect the feet, as in cases of graft-versus-host disease, and the Foot Clinic should be aware of side-effects of surgery, chemotherapy and radiotherapy.

It is also important to look out for possible malignancies affecting other parts of the body in patients who come to the Foot Clinic. When in doubt, always refer onwards is an important maxim. It is difficult to differentiate between benign and malignant conditions without a biopsy, and sometimes several biopsies may be needed to confirm the diagnosis. This chapter discusses squamous cell lesions, melanoma, haematological malignancies, basal cell lesions and differential diagnosis.

Squamous cell lesions

8.1 Squamous cell carcinoma. This lady had a small brown nodule on the sole of her foot and applied a proprietary verucca cure. The lesion ulcerated and became very painful. She went to her general practitioner who diagnosed diabetes. The lesion was initially thought to be a diabetic foot ulcer, but she had no neuropathy and no ischaemia. This is a squamous cell carcinoma, diagnosed after biopsy by the Dermatology Department.

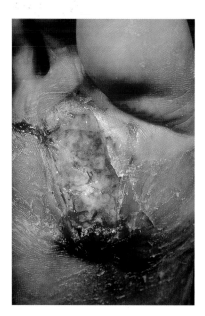

8.2 Squamous cell carcinoma. This is a squamous cell carcinoma, which arose within the scar from a partial amputation of the hallux performed 6 years previously.

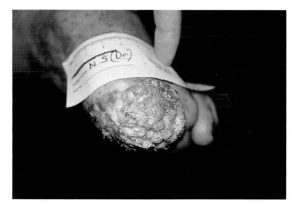

8.3 Squamous cell carcinoma. This ulcer has arisen in a surgical scar. Malignancy should be suspected when old scars, or chronic injuries and ulcers fail to progress.

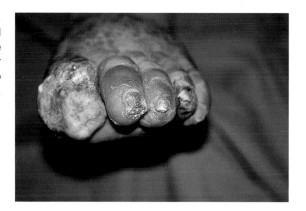

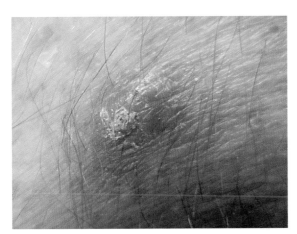

8.4 Squamous cell carcinoma. This lesion arose de novo on the lower leg of a patient with a renal transplant. Patients with transplants are very prone to develop skin malignancy.

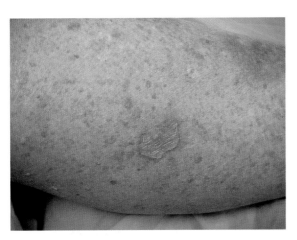

8.5 Excision of squamous cell carcinoma. The lesion has been excised and grafted. The patient needs to be followed up very frequently.

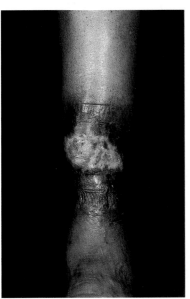

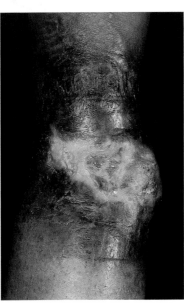

A   **B**

8.6A Suspected malignancy in old yaws scar. This patient was born in Jamaica and lived there until the age of 40. As a child he suffered from yaws, a tropical infection leading to raspberry-like lesions and chronic ulceration. This was treated with antibiotics and the ulcers healed. However, 20 years later he developed this indolent lesion in the scar and was referred by the Foot Clinic to the Dermatology Department. Biopsy revealed a squamous cell carcinoma. **8.6B** Close-up view of same lesion. The squamous cell carcinoma was excised and grafted.

8.7 Cauliflower-like growth. This patient with diabetes underwent debridement and amputation of the toes for severe infection. Many years later this cauliflower-like growth developed on the foot. It was only after three biopsies on three different occasions that the diagnosis of squamous cell carcinoma was obtained.

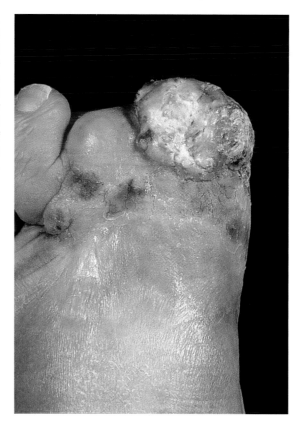

Melanoma

8.8 Malignant melanoma. This is an amelanotic malignant melanoma, which was initially thought to be a subungual exostosis. The toe was amputated and there was no recurrence.

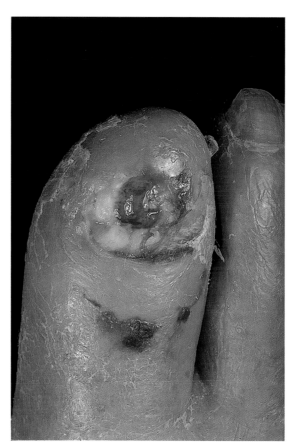

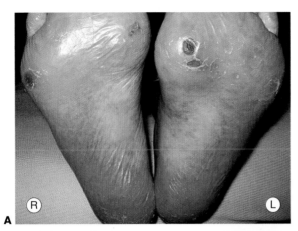

A

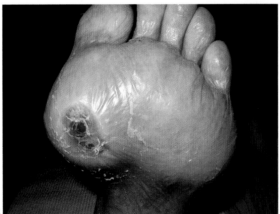

B

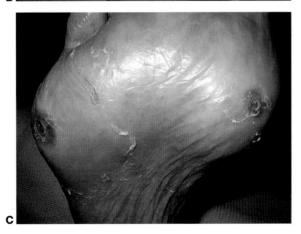

C

8.9A Graft-versus-host disease. This is a reaction of immuno-competent donor cells against the tissues of an immuno-incompetent host. It occurs in patients treated with bone-marrow transplant. These are the feet of a patient with chronic graft-versus-host disease, who has developed ulceration and necrosis on pressure areas of the soles of the feet. The skin is red and painful.
8.9B Graft-versus-host disease: close-up view of ulceration of the left foot.
8.9C Ulcerations on the right foot of the same patient.

8.10 Mycosis fungoides. This patient has a cutaneous T-cell lymphoma which has invaded the skin, giving rise to the painful and unpleasant condition also known as mycosis fungoides. There is grossly increased turnover of skin cells, leading to hyperkeratosis, cracking and ulceration. The texture of the hyperkeratosis is grainy, like Parmesan cheese (due to the presence of micro-abscesses), and has a characteristic mealy odour. Two toes have been amputated due to ulceration and infection, and the wound is not healing. The feet were very painful. In order to keep the patient as comfortable as possible, the podiatrist needed to debride the feet every day, as the patient was unable to walk if they were left for longer. Within 24 hours of debridement, all of the hyperkeratosis had regrown, and a podiatry service was needed at weekends as well as weekdays.

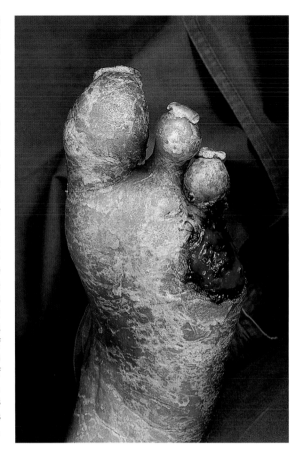

Basal cell lesions

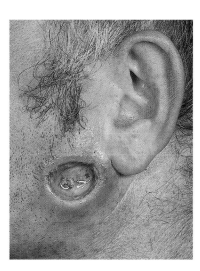

8.11 Neglected basal cell carcinoma (rodent ulcer). This is a suspicious ulcer with a raised, rolled edge on the face of a middle-aged man who lived alone. It was not painful and he never sought treatment. When treating the feet, attention should always be paid to other parts of the body as well. This man was referred to the Dermatology Department after his first appointment at the Foot Clinic: the ulcer was a malignant basal cell carcinoma which was excised. He needed a skin graft. If the ulcer had been reported earlier, then cryotherapy or radiotherapy would have been a feasible treatment. These lesions do not metastasize but can be very locally destructive.

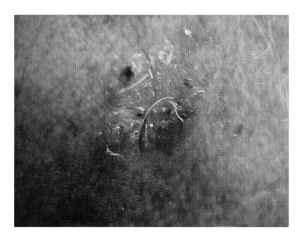

8.12 Basal cell carcinoma. This lesion developed on the dorsum of the foot. The patient did not want to be referred to the Dermatology Department and said he was sure that the problem was trivial; however, he eventually agreed, and the biopsy revealed a basal cell carcinoma, which was treated with cryotherapy.

Differential diagnosis

8.13 Malignancy or extravasation? Malignant lesions can sometimes be difficult to differentiate from callus with old extravasation, as in this case, which occurred on the rocker bottom of a Charcot foot on a site of chronic ulceration. This patient had an indolent neuropathic ulcer, which was debrided at fortnightly intervals. The patient was found to have a darkened area of tissue, which had developed very rapidly. The differential diagnosis of this pigmented lesion was either a malignant melanoma or an area of haemorrhage within the soft tissue. The lesion was referred to the pigmented lesion clinic of the Dermatology Department and biopsied. No melanoma was found. If there is any doubt, patients should be referred to the Dermatology Department without delay.

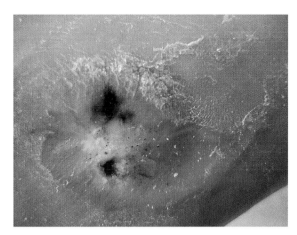

8.14 Pigmented nail band. This patient was referred to the pigmented lesion clinic at the Dermatology Department and underwent biopsy to exclude a malignant melanoma.

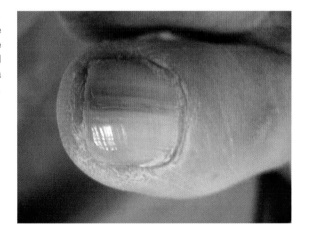

Dermatological conditions

Introduction

Dermatological conditions give rise to many foot problems. This chapter covers specific complications of the skin which are seen in the foot. They include dry skin, corns and callus, neuropathic ulcers, verrucae, pressure ulcers, dermatitis artifacta, traumatic injuries, immersion injuries, thermal injuries, skin grafts, contact dermatitis, varicose (stasis) dermatitis and various other skin conditions. Finally, there is a discussion of maggot therapy for foot ulceration.

9

Dry skin

9.1A Dry callus and fissuring. The skin on the left heel of this patient is dry and fragile. The patient used to soak his feet in the bath for long periods, which exacerbated the dryness. He was advised to use an emollient twice daily.

9.1B Fissures. The right heel has developed deep fissures. Regular application of an emollient will render the dry skin more flexible and prevent fissuring.

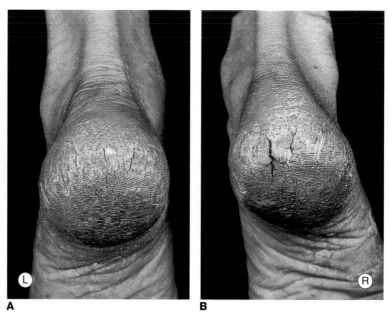

A   B

9.2 Dry skin. This is excessively dry skin in a diabetic patient with neuropathy.

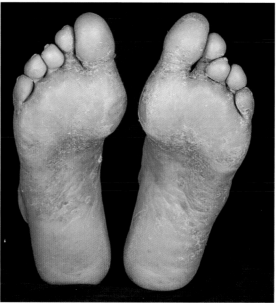

9.3 Dry skin and dermal fissures. This diabetic patient failed to seek treatment for his dry skin and has developed a deep dermal fissure. This was treated by debridement of callus to clear the edges of the fissure, which were then held together with steristrips. Once closed, emollient was applied daily and the problem did not recur.

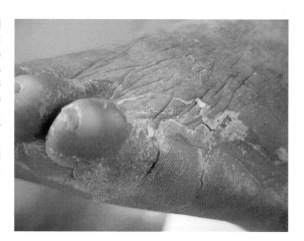

Corns and callus

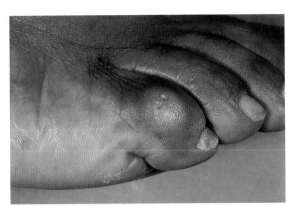

9.4 Callus on a toe. This has formed in response to pressure from a shoe with a very narrow toe box. This toe was subjected to pressure from "winkle picker" shoes. As a reaction, the toe has become inflamed and developed callus.

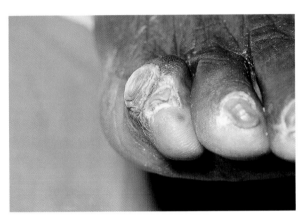

9.5 Heloma durum, a hard corn. When callus is neglected, corns develop. Note the dark halo of post-inflammatory hyperpigmentation at the proximal margin of the corn. When sharp debriding corns that are so close to the nail plate, it can be difficult for the podiatrist to differentiate between what is corn and what is nail.

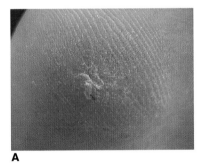

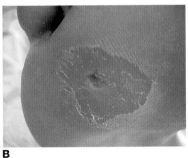

A **B**

9.6A Corn. A corn is an area of callus that is deeper than surrounding callus, and is usually found on the site of highest pressure. The correct treatment is by sharp debridement where every part of the corn is removed. **9.6B** The corn has been dissected out. The telltale signs of increased pressure on underlying tissues from the corn can be seen, with leaking of blood from capillaries and a rim of whitish macerated tissue. Following debridement, the shoes should be adapted or changed to avoid further pressure or friction upon the site.

9.7A Callus pre-debridement. Heavy, neglected callus on the plantar surface of the foot over the 4th and 5th metatarsal head is causing damage to the underlying soft tissues. Note the dark area of haemorrhage and the sinus within the callus where exudate is draining. This plaque of dry callus on the plantar surface of a neuropathic foot thus reveals the tell-tale sign of unacceptably high pressure – bleeding within the callus. The callus must be removed to prevent an ulcer from developing.

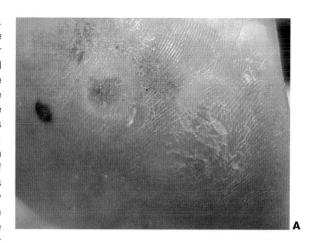

9.7B Callus post debridement. The callus has been removed to reveal maceration and an ulcer. If infection is controlled and pressure relieved this will heal quickly. Off-loading the area to prevent callus formation will be an essential part of future management and this can be achieved with suitable footwear and insole. A suitable insole to reduce plantar pressure to the site will help to prevent further callus formation.

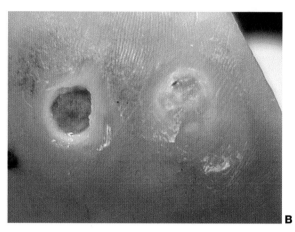

9.8 Hyperkeratosis. This patient has hyperkeratosis. The plaque of callus on the plantar surface consists of yellowish material. If this is allowed to dry out there will be danger of fissuring; regular application of emollients, preferably on a daily basis, will help to prevent this.

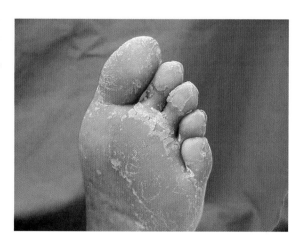

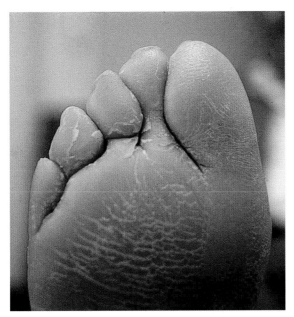

9.9 Benign familial hereditary hyperkeratosis. A rare case of benign familial hyperkeratosis in an elderly male patient. Both the palms and the soles of the feet were affected. In his family tree, his paternal grandfather, one of his two uncles and both his sons had similar problems, but no female relatives were affected. He was seen every month when the edges of cracks in the hyperkeratosis were removed together with flaps of keratin. If this was not performed he quickly developed painful fissures extending into the dermis, and constantly traumatized his feet when flaps of skin became enmeshed in his socks and were torn when the socks were removed.

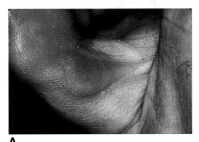

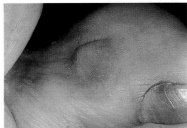

A　　　　　　　　　　**B**

9.10A Soft corn. This lesion is a soft corn, caused by pressure from a prominent interphalangeal joint on the adjoining toe.
9.10B Soft corn. Oblique view of the same lesion.

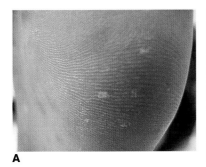

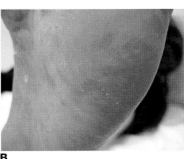

A　　　　　　　　　　**B**

9.11A Seed corns. These lesions are heloma miliare, also called seed corns. They are common in patients with dry skin, and may become painful. They can be easily debrided with a scalpel. Regular application of an emollient to affected areas is useful. **9.11B** The seed corns have been debrided with a scalpel.

9.12A Callus with sinus.
9.12B Post-operative view of the same foot.

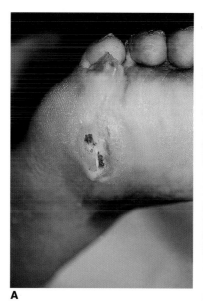

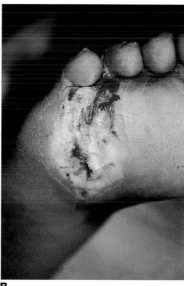

A

B

Neuropathic ulcer

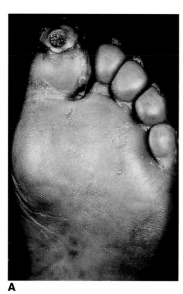

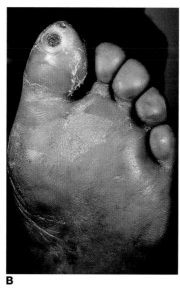

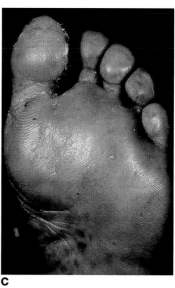

A

B

C

9.13A Neuropathic ulcer on the apex of the hallux. The ulcer was detected at a routine appointment at the diabetic clinic. This Afro-Caribbean woman had no complaints about her feet but was asked to remove her shoes by the physician. **9.13B** Same foot, 1 month later. The ulcer has been treated with antibiotics and weekly sharp debridement by the podiatrist and the orthotist has provided special shoes. The ulcer is smaller and the callus is well controlled. **9.13C** After 2 more weeks the ulcer is fully healed. The patient continued to wear her special shoes and attend the Foot Clinic regularly for callus removal and nail care and remained ulcer-free for many years.

Verrucae

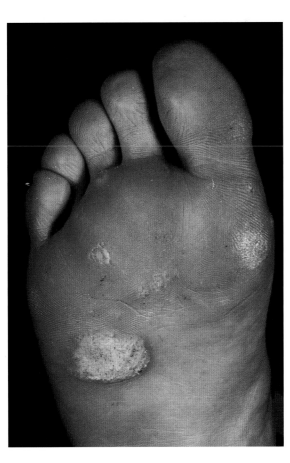

9.14 Verrucae. These plantar warts are sharply defined lesions with hyperkeratotic surface. It is sometimes difficult to distinguish them from corns. Warts are painful when squeezed, while corns are painful when pressed.

9.15A Verrucae. These lesions have a rough warty surface.
9.15B Initial treatment of verrucae. The lesions have been gently debrided and a protective pressure pad applied.
9.15C Close-up of verrucae after treatment.

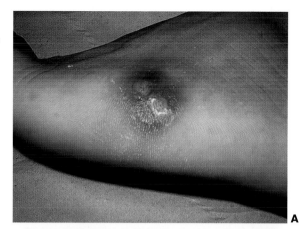

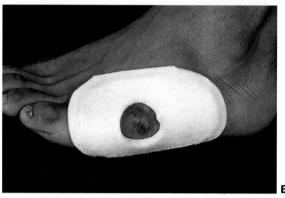

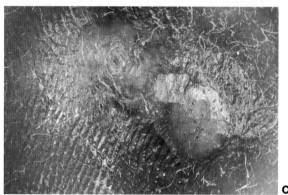

Pressure ulcer

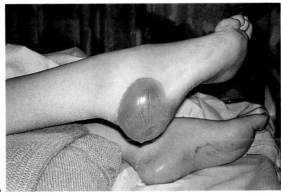

A

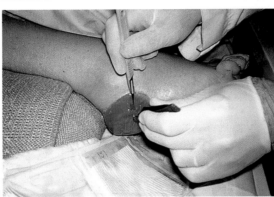

B

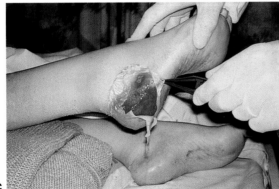

C

9.16A Pressure ulcer. This elderly, frail lady was admitted with a stroke. Once on the ward, her heel was noted to be red and was immediately protected with a foam wedge, but she developed a large heel bulla in response to a previous period of unrelieved pressure. **9.16B** The podiatrist is puncturing the blister with a scalpel to relieve hydrostatic pressure. **9.16C** The blister is being deroofed. It is now possible to inspect the base.

Dermatitis artifacta

9.17 Picking heel: self-inflicted injury. This patient has injured her heel by pulling off pieces of loose skin. She found it a difficult habit to overcome, especially in the evenings if she was watching television, when she would curl up on a sofa without her shoes on. She found that wearing white cotton socks in the evenings helped her to resist temptation.

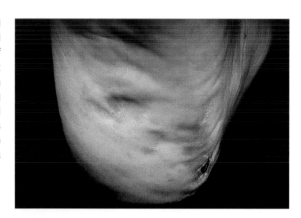

9.18 Picking off skin and causing ulcer. This patient is 29 years old and has been diabetic since the age of 3 years. She is a known case of dermatitis artifacta, with numerous hospital admissions for infected wounds. This lesion was caused by failure to apply an emollient to dry skin, and picking and pulling pieces of skin off.

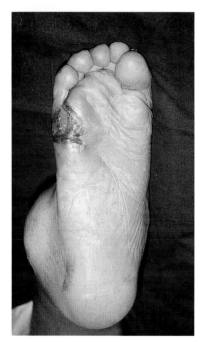

9.19 Dermatitis artifacta in a diabetic patient with neuropathy. This lesion was caused by soaking a small dressing in lavatory cleaner and applying it to the dorsum of the foot. It is a hard condition to diagnose. Look out for the warning signs; the condition is often seen in patients with a history of eating disorders and patients who work as health-care professionals. Patients frequently present with strange lesions that may have unusual morphology (straight edges), unusual sites, or no explanation of how the lesions occurred.

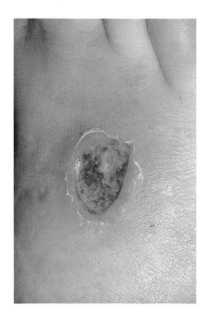

Traumatic injuries

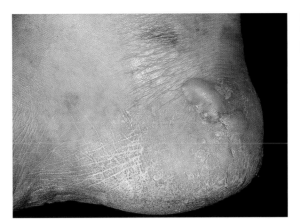

9.20 Heel fissure and blister. This was secondary to a shoe injury.

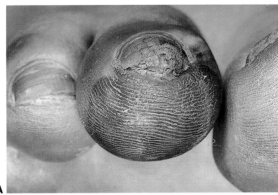

A

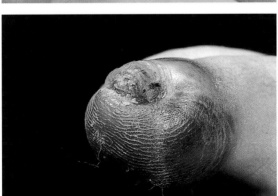

B

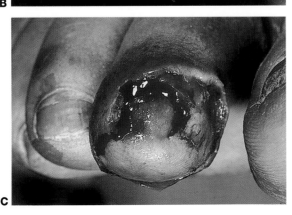

C

9.21A Blood blister. The patient did not know the cause of the injury as there was an underlying neuropathy, but examination revealed a ruckled shoe lining that had rubbed the toe.
9.21B Side view of the toe reveals a very tense, bulging blood blister, which had a very hard consistency on palpation.
9.21C The blood blister has been drained and deroofed: it incorporated the entire nail plate, which was floating on a bed of sanguinous fluid and has been removed to enable full inspection and drainage. The toe healed in 2 weeks. The patient was advised to check his shoes regularly, to shake them out before wearing them, and to run his hand around the inside of the shoes to detect any rough places.

Immersion injuries

9.22A "Trench foot". This is "trench foot", so named because it was common among soldiers in the trenches of the First World War. Trench foot is an immersion injury. This patient had been working in her garden wearing leaky Wellington boots, and muddy water seeped into the boots. Her skin became macerated and the skin was abraded by the wet lining and the gritty consistency of the mud.

9.22B A closer view of the same foot. See the transverse fissuring as the foot dries out. She needed tetanus prophylaxis.

9.22C Trench foot. This patient was a swimming instructor who had also developed tinea pedis. The vesicles on the 1st toe coalesced to form a large bulla, which became macerated in the pool and ruptured when she walked on the tiles at the side of the pool.

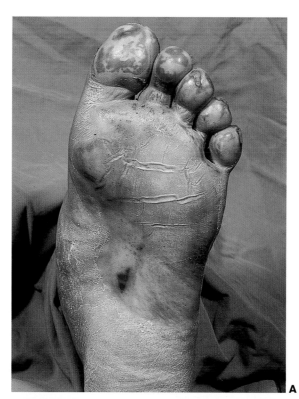

A

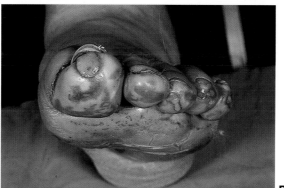

B

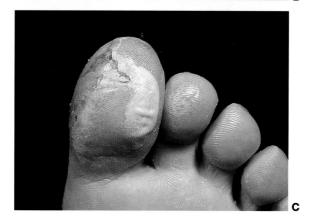

C

Thermal injuries

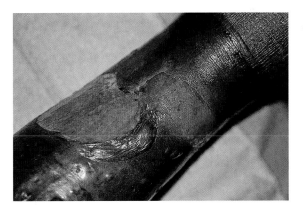

9.23 Burn on leg from hot fat. This Afro-Caribbean patient burned his leg when he dropped a chip pan and splashed himself with hot fat. He was referred to a specialist burns unit.

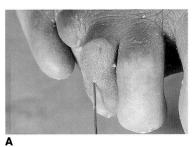
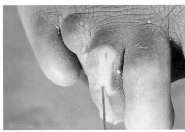

A   **B**

9.24A Burn blister management. A narrow gauge hypodermic needle has been inserted to drain the small, tense bulla on the dorsum of the 3rd toe. The adjoining toe was amputated the previous year after a similar bulla on the 4th toe became infected.

9.24B The bulla is now flaccid. Fluid has been sent to the laboratory for microscopy and culture.

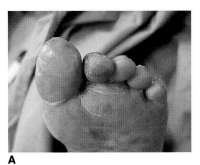
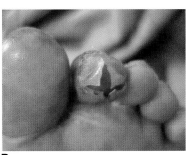

A   **B**

9.25A Burn blister with blue discolouration from hydrostatic pressure. Patients with neuropathy frequently burn their feet inadvertently and should be warned never to use hot-water bottles or apply other forms of heat directly to the feet. Neuropathic patients often have the sensation that their feet are cold. This patient toasted his toes in front of a fan heater. He has a severe burn on the apex of the 2nd toe, which is blistered and discoloured.

9.25B A cross cut is made in the burn to expose the base. The wound bed has become pink after the contents of the blister were evacuated, thus relieving the hydrostatic pressure and enabling the wound bed to be inspected.

9.26A Blister management. This patient presented with a large blister involving the heel and the arch of the foot. He did not know the cause, although it may have been a thermal injury. He had alcoholic neuropathy, lacked protective pain sensation and frequently walked barefoot. It is inevitable that a blister of this size will eventually rupture. If the fluid contents are tense this may cause necrosis and it is, therefore, important to inspect the base of the blister. If this large lesion becomes infected it will be a very serious problem. A cross has been cut in the blister for drainage and inspection. **9.26B** The quadrants of the cross-cut blister can be lifted back for inspection. The wound bed is pink and clean. **9.26C** The quadrants have been folded back over the wound bed. There is a chance that the epithelial cells on the underside may adhere, survive and grow, thus achieving very rapid closure.

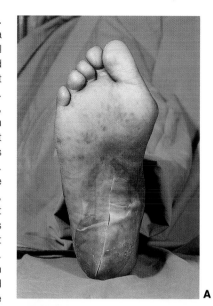

A

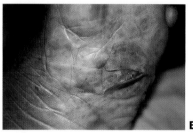

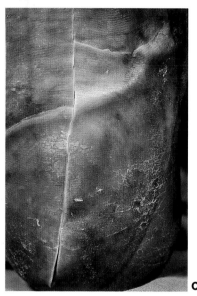

B

C

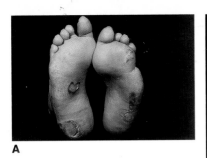

A

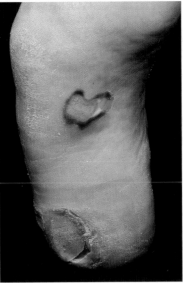

B

9.27A Burns from foot spa. This patient was a neuropathic patient with diabetes. He frequently complained of paraesthesiae in his feet, and his wife bought him a foot spa. In these devices the feet are soaked in vibrating, hot water, which caused severe injuries in this case. Patients with peripheral neuropathy should be advised never to use a foot spa. **9.27B** Close-up view of burnt right foot from foot spa.

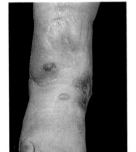

A

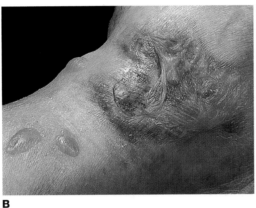

B

9.28A Burnt foot from fan heater. This 77-year-old lady with diabetes, who had previously lost part of her 2nd toe because of ischaemic gangrene, sustained these burns when she sat too close to a convector heater. **9.28B** Close-up view of the medial aspect of the foot of the same patient.

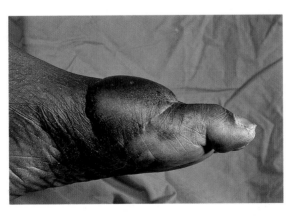

9.29 Huge bulla from spilled tea. This Afro-Caribbean patient with neuropathy developed a large bulla. She was not aware of having traumatized the foot, but later remembered having dropped a cup of hot tea. The blister was drained and the foot healed within 2 weeks.

9.30 Full-thickness sunburn. This is a full-thickness burn on the dorsum of the foot, sustained by a patient who had lain on the beach and fallen asleep.

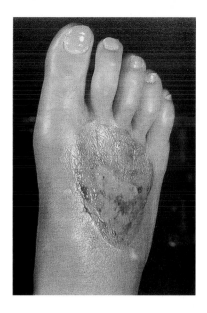

Skin grafts

9.31A Split skin graft. This Afro-Caribbean patient with a dorsal "phlegmon" underwent debridement and skin grafting. There is post-inflammatory hyperpigmentation in the foot, so the graft, which was taken from the patient's thigh, looks very pale in contrast. In the early days many successful grafts may look non-viable but should not be removed until it is certain that they have not taken.

9.31B Close-up view of the same foot. There is an erosion on the graft that will need to heal by secondary intention.

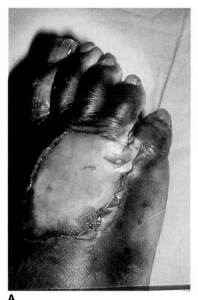

A

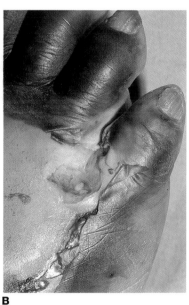

B

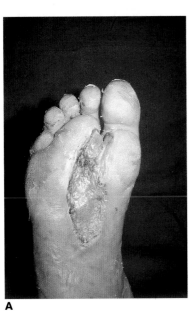

A

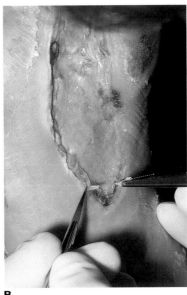

B

9.32A Skin graft with border hyperkeratosis. Debriding callus from around a skin graft can help to prevent ulceration and loss of grafted tissue, and long-term management of pedal skin grafts in patients with neuropathy is an important aspect of foot care. This patient underwent split-skin grafting to a large tissue defect following an episode of severe infection. The graft is growing callus 2 months later, which will require regular debridement by the podiatrist. Special shoes with cradled insoles will also help to offload excessive pressure on the skin graft. **9.32B** The podiatrist is sharp debriding hyperkeratosis from the skin graft of the patient.

Contact dermatitis

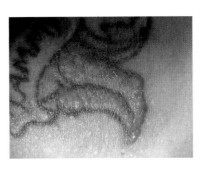

9.33 Tattoo allergy. This patient developed an allergic contact dermatitis to the red dye in a tattoo on the side of his foot. Allergy to red dye is very common and may occur immediately or, as in this case, may be delayed.

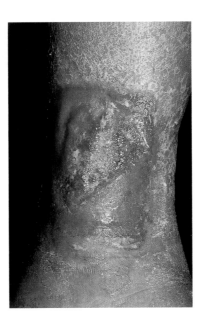

9.34 Contact dermatitis to foam dressing. This patient developed contact dermatitis involving the precise area covered by a foam dressing. He removed the dressing and scratched the area. Patients with venous eczema frequently have hypersensitive skin that reacts badly to dressings. This patient was allergic to all foam and hydrocolloid dressings.

9.35 Secondary infection of contact dermatitis. This patient reacted to a dressing and developed a contact dermatitis but did not regard it as serious until the area became secondarily infected. The infection required systemic antibiotics and took several weeks to heal. There was underlying venous disease and healing was difficult to achieve.

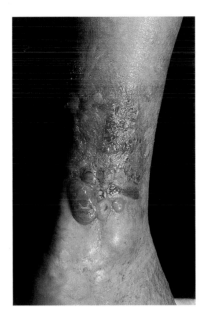

9.36 Contact dermatitis with resolving secondary infection.

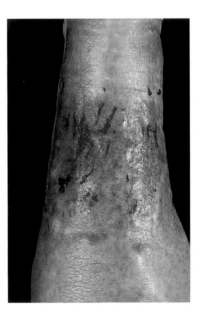

9.37 Dermatitis following topical antibiotic ointment. This patient applied topical antibiotic ointment to a painful crack on the side of the toe and developed an allergic reaction with severe dermatitis in the area where the ointment had been applied.

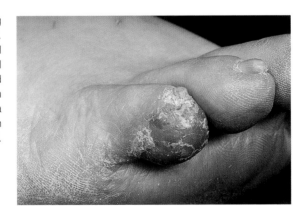

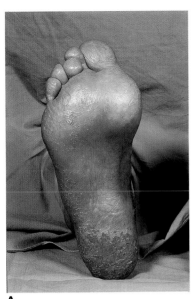

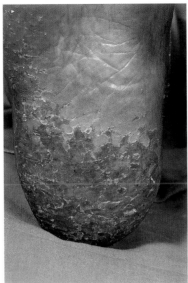

A   **B**

9.38A Dermatitis caused by foam heel cup. This patient developed painful fissuring on the heel and was wearing a foam heel cup. He developed a contact dermatitis affecting the precise area covered by the dressing. **9.38B** Close-up view of same patient.

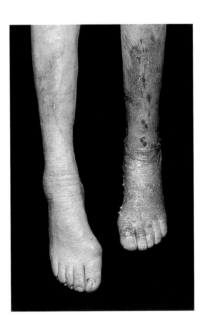

9.39 Dermatitis caused by allergy to biological washing powder. This patient developed dermatitis with rash and itching, which was first thought to be a fungal infection. The problem did not resolve with topical antifungal agents and the laboratory was unable to observe or culture fungus from skin scrapings. The problem began after his wife started to use a biological washing powder and resolved after she reverted to the former powder used.

Varicose (Stasis) dermatitis

9.40A Varicose dermatitis. This patient had neglected varicose (stasis) eczema with crusting. The scaly crusted lesions are greasy and waxy, and if allowed to become too thick there will be a risk of breakdown of the underlying tissues.

9.40B The thicker scales have been carefully removed with forceps. Note the underlying hypopigmentation and maceration.

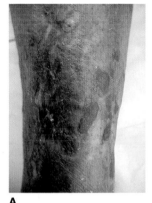
A

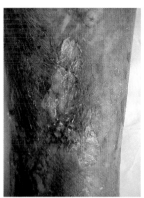
B

9.41 Eczematous stasis dermatitis. The patient had chronic venous insufficiency complicated by inflammation of the lower legs presenting as an eczematous stasis dermatitis. It is often misdiagnosed as cellulitis.

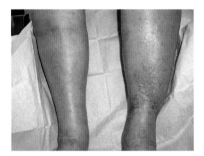

9.42 Erythematous rash with pustules. This was caused by a secondary staphyloccal infection in a patient with pre-existing venous insufficiency, chronic stasis dermatitis and oedema.

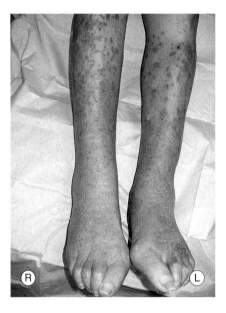

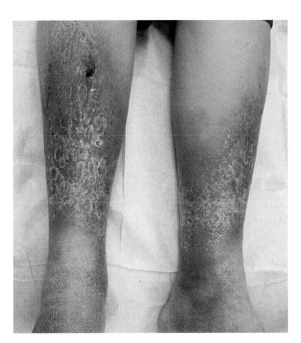

9.43 Eczematous stasis dermatitis with inflammation and scaling.

Miscellaneous skin conditions

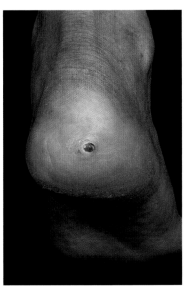

A

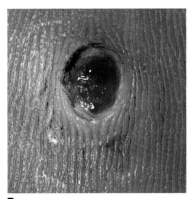

B

9.44A Eccrine poroma. This is a solitary benign tumour.
9.44B Close-up of the same lesion. The lesion is well defined and has a sessile base.

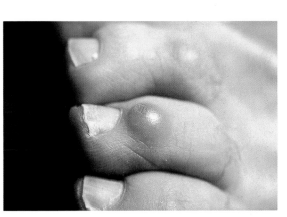

9.45 Adventitious bursa. This patient has a deformed toe. This deformity has subjected the toe to pressure from the toe box of the shoe, leading to formation of a small adventitious bursa over the dorsal interphalangeal joint.

9.46 Vasculitis. This painful ulcer developed from a haemorrhagic pustule. There was a purple red margin to the ulcer, which was complicated by necrotic eschar. The patient responded to topical steroid therapy.

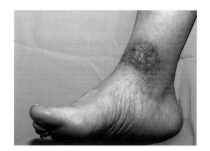

9.47A Vasculitis. There were multiple ulcerated lesions on the lower legs associated with lower limb and ankle oedema. These lesions responded to steroid therapy. **9.47B** Extensive ulceration on posterior aspect of lower leg.

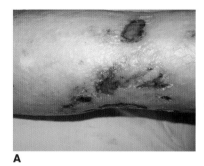

A

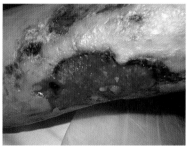

B

9.48 Differential diagnosis. Vasculitic lesions or emboli? This diabetic patient developed discrete palpable lesions on the feet. He had peripheral vascular disease with occlusive arterial disease of the iliac and femoral arteries, but the biopsy showed leucocytoclastic vasculitis.

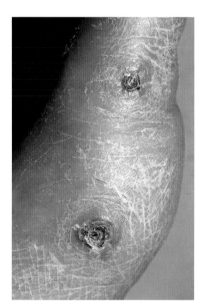

9.49 A right red foot and leg. A problem of differential diagnosis. Questioning elicited the information that the patient was an amateur bee keeper who had been stung by a tray of bees that had been dropped down his Wellington boot!

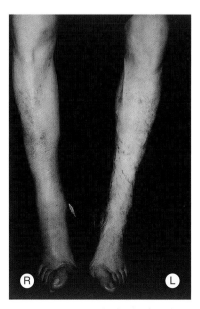

Maggot therapy

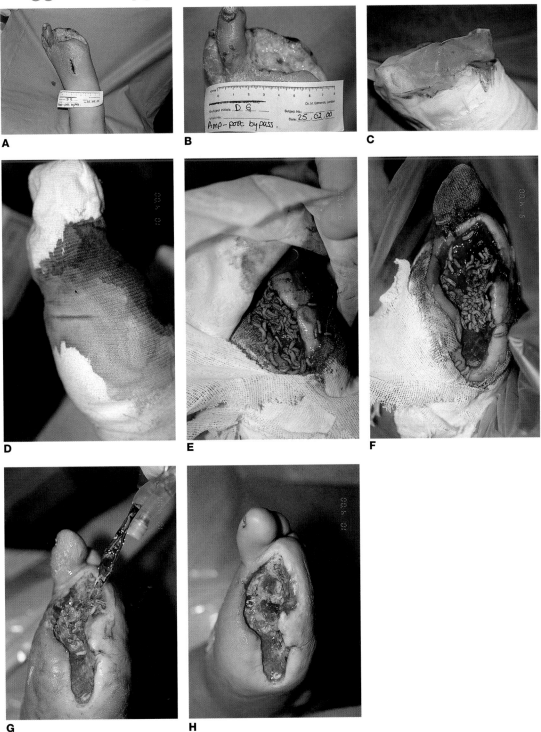

9.50A Maggot therapy. This patient with diabetes and peripheral vascular disease underwent distal bypass and amputation of three toes. The wound soon became very sloughy. **9.50B** Close-up of the wound. Antibiotics were prescribed. **9.50C** Sterile medical maggots of L. Sericata were obtained from a medical maggot supplier and applied to the wound. They were contained within a special fine mesh cage, as shown here. The normal skin surrounding the wound was masked with calorband. The foot was then dressed with moistened saline gauze and a light bandage. The gauze was not saturated with fluid and the bandage was loose because of the danger that the very small and immature maggots might suffocate or drown. **9.50D** One day later the gauze dressing and bandage were soaked in exudate. Maggots produce enzymes in large quantities. **9.50E** The cage is opened to reveal maggots wriggling in the wound. **9.50F** One day later some of the maggots have their pointed heads down and their blunt tails exposed: a sign that they are feeding. They are much less active. **9.50G** On the 4th day the maggots are no longer feeding and are irrigated out of the wound with a jet of sterile water. **9.50H** A close-up view of the wound reveals that the maggots have removed much of the slough.

9.51 A wild maggot.

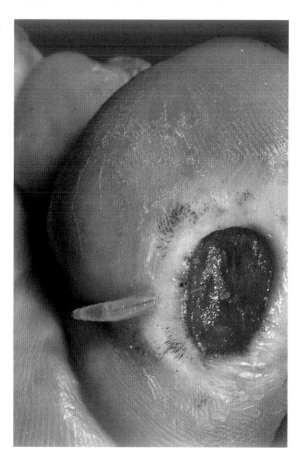